Nutrition in Focus

Nutrition in Focus

Sonia Jones

Zambezi Publishing Ltd

First published in 2023 in the UK by Zambezi Publishing Ltd
Plymouth, Devon PL2 2EQ
Tel: +44 (0)1752 367 300
email: zambezipub@gmail.com   www.zampub.com

British Library Cataloguing in Publication Data:
A catalogue record for this book is available from the British Library

ISBN(13) 978-1-903065-98-3
Illustrations copyright © 2023
Jan Budkowski, Dreamstime.com
Typesetting by Zambezi Publishing Ltd, Plymouth

Disclaimer:- This book is intended to provide general information
regarding the subject matter, and to entertain. The contents are not
exhaustive and no warranty is given as to accuracy of content. The book
is sold on the understanding that neither the publisher nor the author
are thereby engaged in rendering professional services, in respect of the
subject matter or any other field. If expert guidance is required, the
services of a qualified professional should be sought.
Readers are urged to access a range of other material on the book's
subject matter, and to tailor the information to their individual needs.
Neither the author nor the publisher shall have any responsibility to any
person or entity regarding any loss or damage caused or alleged to be
caused, directly or indirectly, by the use or misuse of information
contained in this book. If you do not wish to be bound by the above,
you may return this book in original condition to the publisher, with its
receipt, for a refund of the purchase price.

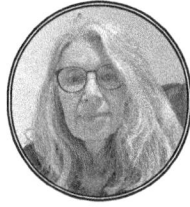

About the Author

Sonia Jones is a Naturopath and Nutritional Therapist who trained in Australia and England. She has spent many years in the health and hospitality business, a business she recently sold. On returning to the UK, Sonia has made the West Country her permanent home, together with her dog, Holly. Sonia makes all her dog's food - it's totally natural.

Her days are spent writing and working on a new venture called Cwtch Lifestyle (https://cwtchlifestyle.com). She has been an advocate of a healthy natural diet and a sustainable lifestyle for several decades, and advocated upcycling long before it became popular. Sonia knows that good nutrition is truly fundamental to a healthy life, and hopes that this book will help people achieve the best lifestyle possible for themselves.

Contents

Introduction

Nutrition is a process by which we take on board and utilise plant and animal food substances. Digestion breaks this food down into components, which is a substantial daily undertaking. I would say that most of us take this for granted until something goes wrong. We only worry about our digestion if we suffer from heartburn, constipation, diarrhoea, trapped wind, nausea, feeling hungry all the time, cravings, bloating, feeling tired after eating, uncomfortable or even in pain. Many adults suffer from these problems, and while they may not be life threatening, they can be lifestyle threatening, and in the long run, these symptoms can lead to severe conditions.

We need to obtain certain things from our foods, including protein, fat, carbohydrates, vitamins, minerals, enzymes, water and electrolytes. We all know this, but do we think about it when we eat and drink? And do we consider how our choices might impact upon us?

We are all different, and we all have a different genetic makeup, so this might lead one person to suffer from one ailment and another person to suffer from something else. It may even have some effect on your body size and shape. However, we may overlook eating habits that we picked up in childhood, and we may put ailments that affect various family members down to genetic factors when they actually come, in part at least, from an inherited eating pattern. Some ailments run in families, with type-2 diabetes being an obvious one, but even this ailment can be controlled to a great extent by keeping to a sensible diet. Diabetes is on the increase, and much (although not all) of this is due to obesity.

The media is happy to write things that interest the public, but not all of this is actually useful, and some things are confusing. We are told to count calories, and then not to count calories, or that we should eat spread in place of butter or that we should not eat spread in place of butter. We are told that alcohol is good for us or it is destructive, that we should eat more protein or less of it, that we should cut the carbs, eat eggs, not eat eggs and so on. Much of this misleading information comes from the food industry, which has vested interests in what they tell us.

So, if research has revealed that the rate at which we age is genetically predetermined, why should we worry? Why should we bother? Let us just eat, drink and be merry. Or, we could take another view, which is to make the most of what we have been given, so let us try and make sure we do everything possible to make our lives as happy, healthy, active and pain-free as possible.

If we consider anything worth having, it's usually something we have to pursue actively. Where health is concerned, few of us live on junk food, drink too much and then expect to live a long and happy life. Most of us would like to think we could do whatever we like and then pop a few multivitamins and minerals or an antacid or have a session at the gym and remain energetic, fit and healthy. However, those of you who are prepared to make a few lifestyle changes will reap huge, long and short term benefits.

Introduction

This book will help you to achieve benefits in a simple and achievable way, as there are no agonising exercises to do, no calorie counting, no drugs and no concoctions to take! It's just sensible nutrition.

> It used to be rare to find young people with adult-onset Diabetes, but they now appear at an alarming rate!

1: Nutrition and Health

1: Nutrition and Health

It would be fair to say that most of us take our health for granted until something goes wrong, and this is a shame because prevention is always easier than trying to fix the problem when it arises. As the saying goes, "You don't know what you've got until it's gone," which is true of our health.

Our requirements for health are pretty straightforward - fresh air, pure drinking water, sunshine and good quality nutrient-rich "live" food. I'm sure you would agree that these are well-being essentials. However, most people consider coffee, chocolate and bread essential. I come across very few people who drink enough water, let alone eat much in the way of live, fresh, enzyme-rich foods.

What do I mean by live, fresh, enzyme-rich foods? Take, for example, two sunflower seeds and boil just one of them, then plant both in the same fertile soil, water them and wait for them to germinate. Only one of the sunflower seeds will burst into life due to the still intact, live enzymes. The seed heated at a high temperature has had its enzymes destroyed, so was unable to germinate and burst into life.

People say that eating healthily is too expensive, but healthy eating doesn't have to be more expensive. Of course, eating healthy food doesn't guarantee that you will never be sick, but it will reduce the odds, and it should reduce the severity or duration of any illnesses. Eating well gives you more energy and a better quality of life. We can choose whether to eat nutrient-poor or nutrient-rich foods - both are easy to find. Nutrient-rich foods are natural foods with little or no processing, unlike nutrient-poor foods.

The food industry will spend a huge budget on advertising their products in a favourable light. Advertising can be very sophisticated and it's convincing. After all, we are all very busy, and they provide such convenience for us, and in some cases, addictive foods. Once you get used to preparing fresh food, it doesn't take that much effort, and after eating well for a while, you will have gained more energy to want to cook more. There is a great sense of pride and well-being in eating food you have prepared that hasn't come from a factory. On this note, there are other considerations to think about, such as the extra packaging and travelling of these convenience foods that take their toll on our environment.

There is the idea that we can get away with not eating so well if we pop a vitamin or two. I wish things were that easy. It should be noted that vitamins and minerals are called supplements because they supplement a healthy diet, so they should not be used instead of a healthy diet. Manufactured vitamins and minerals are second best; they are more difficult to absorb and utilise than the vitamins and minerals from food. Many compounds in natural foods have not yet been researched or are too difficult to replicate and put into a capsule or tablet. Nature provides nutrients in such complex, unique combinations.

A memory came to mind when a good friend told their child who was eating a sausage from their BBQ, "Don't feed that junk to the dog!" Why was it okay for his child to eat that junk if it wasn't good enough for the dog? It's time to re-evaluate what nutrition, food and diet mean to you and your quality of life.

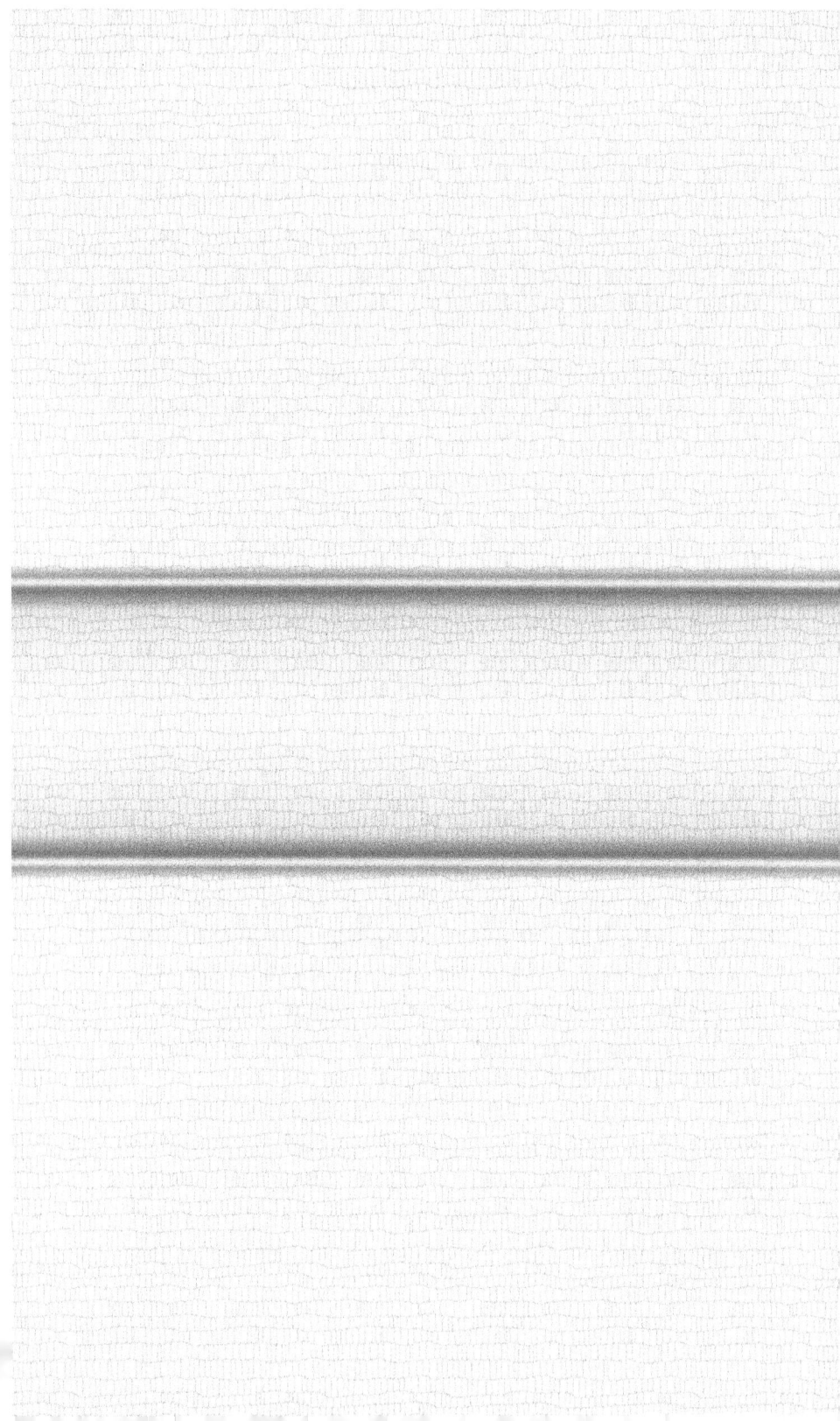

2: Science and Nutrition

2: Science and Nutrition

Evidence backs up the idea that the type of foods we choose to eat has a profound and fundamental impact on the way we deteriorate, and this has far more profound, more far-reaching consequences than the genes we inherited. We can't choose our genes, but we can choose our food and lifestyles.

When we think of health and ageing, we believe it involves some degree of physical and mental decline. However, many people maintain comparatively full physical and mental health throughout a very long life. Nutrition plays a huge part in our physical and psychological well-being, and way too much research has been done to dispute these facts.

Here is an example. I saw a 55-year-old man in our clinic with diabetes, high blood pressure, high cholesterol, poor digestion and heartburn. He was overweight, but this was in a country that did not have a National Health Service, so the biggest worry was that he had been told that further medical insurance might be refused due to his state of health. The amount of surgery he'd already had and the large amounts of medication he was taking were using up his insurance credit. On the other hand, there was a 64-year-old who visited the clinic as part of his maintenance program, and he had none of these problems and was not taking any medication other than vitamins and minerals. He was not overweight and was extremely fit, still riding a bike up and down hills.

No one expects you to buy a mountain bike; I am just pointing out that anything is possible, and you can choose your path. The first man has all the conditions that have generally been proven to be self-inflicted by the lifestyle he chose, and these conditions can improve or even reverse with the right choices.

Incidentally, the first man has made vast improvements in many areas with good nutrition, lifestyle changes and supplements. His recent blood tests have revealed that his bad cholesterol is down, his triglycerides are down, his blood pressure and weight are down and his medication is down. He is a different man, despite having a long way to go.

We are all at risk of not getting adequate nutrients due to the refining and processing of food, but even more so as we get older due to the decline in our digestive function. Fewer calories are needed due to a reduction in general activity. Some older people's appetite declines, partly due to changes or a decline in taste and smell. We may lose our sense of thirst as we age, so dehydration is likely. Our digestive system starts to cause us a problem, having been abused for years.

The stomach slows down its production of digestive juices and enzymes, affecting the absorption of B12, iron and calcium, to name just a few nutrients. There is a reduction in lactase production, which causes milk intolerance. Constipation is often a problem as we age, as more fibre is needed compared to when we were young. Medication can change the way food tastes, cause nausea or affect the way the bowels work. Eating alone can prevent some people from cooking and eating well.

Smoking or vaping robs the body of large amounts of vital nutrients. The list of nutrients needed to repair joint "wear and tear" or maintain healthy bones and teeth is endless. More than just small amounts of alcohol can hurt general health and well-being.

In our culture, we hear of people after a certain age suffering a stroke or arthritis or heart disease, and we hardly bat an eyelid. Yet if we lived in a more traditional society, these diseases would be rare at any age, but very rare at as young an age as now. It would be quite a talking point. For instance, women who eat a traditional diet in Japan hardly ever have osteoporosis, and they have few menopausal symptoms. Yet the modern Japanese women who live on a Western diet now have osteoporosis and the usual symptoms of menopause! This is more to do with their new lifestyle than a sudden gene change. I repeat - it's not those genes!

We need to look at the facts because a speedy decline is not inevitable. So much research proves that things and your life can be different. Your life can be much better, and you can be healthier, happier, slimmer and more active at any stage. Don't be brainwashed by the advertising companies or by the lure of the addictive ingredients sitting on supermarket shelves that are causing chronic problems. Think positively, as starting with healthy nutrition and lifestyle is never too early or too late.

3: Advanced Glycation End Products (AGEs)

3: Advanced Glycation End Products (AGEs)

A particular diet and lifestyle can result in something scary called Advanced Glycation End-products (AGEs); this accelerated destruction is not due to ageing but to your chosen foods and lifestyle. This is a crucial aspect of our long-term health.

Our bodies use glucose as energy converted into other substances through Krebs or citric cycles. This enables the body to utilise it fully. However, our Western diets are overloaded with sugars and refined carbohydrates, alcohol (super sugar) and soft drinks that encourage vast amounts of glucose to enter the bloodstream, causing a huge problem. Our bodies are designed to handle a certain amount of imbalance; we have built-in safety mechanisms for an occasional emergency, but we can't cope with a constant overload which has serious consequences in the long run. This scenario is like a catalyst because we are speeding up the process of our deterioration! This may seem far-fetched, but we are encouraging free-radical damage almost on the scale of smoking or heavy drinking! Excess glucose in our system causes damage to our protein and our very structure.

What does this mean? We are damaging our skin, muscles, organs, brains etc. Our very foundation is being weakened because our cells are being damaged to such an extent that there is cross-linking. This cross-linking speeds up anything from encouraging wrinkled skin to problems with organ function. Damage can occur in any tissue in the body, and impaired organ function can disrupt the delicate balance of hormones, especially those that slow down our body's destruction. The more damage there is, the more is caused, so the situation escalates. It's like a domino effect.

Along with healthy foods, we need our digestive system to be in good working order, and we need plenty of fluids and nutrients to produce enough digestive enzymes. The foods that most people have chosen to eat over the years have been hard to digest, and they supply next to no nutrients needed to break down these foods, let alone enough to service all the other systems in the body.

The Perfect Scenario
Choose to Eat Nutrient-Rich Foods.
Easy-to-digest foods provide nutrients for their digestion, with plenty left over for other functions elsewhere in the body.

What has happened over the years?

- We consume a diet full of refined foods, sugar and poor-quality fats.
- A diet that lacks nutrients and enzymes for the body's digestive process and other processes.
- Digestion struggles and deficiencies are created; hence, more deterioration occurs due to imperfections.

For Instance…
A shortage of zinc affects every aspect of digestion. It affects our taste and smell, and it is noticeable how people

add more and more salt to compensate for the decline in taste and smell.

A zinc deficiency also affects the quality of our hydrochloric acid levels. We need a good supply of zinc for the correct stomach acidity levels.

So Why is this so Important?

- Zinc breaks down calcium to enable us to absorb and utilise it properly.
- Zinc kills bacteria that have entered the body and causes problems.
- Zinc ensures proper protein breakdown.

This is only one nutrient out of many digestion needs required in adequate amounts.

We need plenty of Fluids and Nutrients to produce enough Digestive Enzymes!

4: Digestion

4: Digestion

Enzymes, in general, are a little-discussed aspect of nutrition, but they are vital.

Enzymes act upon substances by changing their original identity, so they are the catalyst. Enzymes are needed for every chemical action and reaction in the body. Metabolic enzymes run everything, encompassing our organs, tissues and cells. Without enzymes, there is no life and no movement. Enzymes are vital to maintaining life. Each enzyme performs a specific job within the body. Some are involved in digestion, while others aid detoxification or are needed for building new bones or skin. Enzymes form urea, aiding the immune system, helping in fertilisation, transporting oxygen around the body, or breaking down old cells. Just about every process in the body needs enzymes.

Machines are lifeless until batteries have been installed or the electricity has been switched on. Enzymes activate a reaction without which we would be dead. Life cannot exist without them.

Where do these enzymes originate? Our body can manufacture enzymes, or they can come from our food. Although the latter statement is correct, most people's food lacks live enzymes and good-quality nutrients. The problem with enzymes is their sensitivity to heat and light. Cooking destroys them, and so do canning, frying, roasting, pasteurising, etc.

4: Digestion

Most foods on supermarket shelves have been subject to high heat levels, their enzymes have been destroyed, and nutrients and fibre have been removed during the manufacturing process. Each time you eat such "empty calories", you have to make enzymes or find the nutrients to digest these foods, causing a deficit somewhere in the body. As time goes on, the situation slowly gets worse.

It has been found that young people have greater reserves of enzymes in their tissues; when a young person eats cooked foods, there is a more significant activity of enzymes than in an older adult. Have you ever wondered why we end up with digestive problems as we age? As our enzyme reserves become depleted over the years, and as we continue to eat "dead food", our digestive system begins to struggle. The gradual depletion of enzymes means that most food isn't being digested properly. For instance, studies have shown low levels of enzymes in people with diabetes. The pancreas is the organ that produces insulin and digestive enzymes. People suffering from liver problems have also been found to have low levels of digestive enzyme activity.

It's common today to find people living on stimulants. When our metabolism is falsely stimulated with caffeine, alcohol, high-protein diets, chocolate and sugar, enzymes and nutrients are spent, and our reserves are slowly used up. False energy is experienced, and eventually, we become fatigued. It's like using a whip on a horse; it will run faster, but it's not the whip that gives the horse energy; it's the stimulant of pain. We become dependent on these stimulants to function normally. We need more and more to feel normal, leading to premature ageing and chronic diseases.

Vitamins and minerals depend on enzymes, while enzymes depend on vitamins and minerals. Nature has provided us with foods rich in enzymes, vitamins and minerals. Enzymes and nutrients are used much faster than usual during exercise and acute disease (especially fevers and infections). Anything that increases heat in the body will speed up enzyme activity. As you would expect, enzyme activity also goes up during digestion.

There is a direct relationship between our enzyme reserve and the health of our immune system. The better our enzyme reserve, the better our immune system can cope with everyday battles, of which there are many. White blood cells seek out and destroy foreign invaders infiltrating our blood and lymph. Studies have shown that these white blood cells have proteolytic, amylolytic and lipolytic enzymes similar to those produced by the pancreas for digestion. These enzymes break down proteins, fat and carbohydrates that have escaped into the bloodstream, thus dealing with them before they cause too much havoc or destruction in our system.

Digestive Enzymes

We eat three types of food: proteins, carbohydrates and fats, for which there are three primary groups of digestive enzymes.

- Proteolytic enzymes break down proteins into amino acids, of which there are about twenty-two. Nine of these are called "essential". The body cannot make them, so they need to be provided by the diet. The others can be made within the body.
- Amylolytic enzymes break down carbohydrates.
- Lipolytic enzymes break down fats called lipids.

What Affects Enzymes?

Pesticides, including insecticides, herbicides and fungicides, inhibit enzymes. Fruit and vegetables are sprayed many times during their growing season. Always wash fruit, salad and vegetables to remove sprays, wax and germs. Buy organic produce if you can afford it, or grow your own.

Salt and sugar have been used for centuries to preserve food as they inhibit enzyme activity.

Food additives, of which there are hundreds. They are used by the food industry to make food more palatable and to give foodstuffs a longer shelf life. Who knows what long-term health effects these will have?

Is the Digestive System Struggling?

There are numerous common ailments that many people suffer and are seen as almost a normal part of life:

Heartburn.
Diarrhoea.
Constipation.
Diverticulitis.
Poor sense of smell and taste.
Cravings.
Blood sugar problems.
Weight fluctuations.
Bloating.
Pains.
Piles.
Wind.
Sweating after eating.
Tired after eating.
Fluid retention.
Hiatus Hernia.
Ulcers.
Gall bladder problems.

IBS.
Anaemia.
Feeling always full.
Always hungry.

These ailments can all be improved or even reversed by good nutrition, which will, in turn, improve digestion.

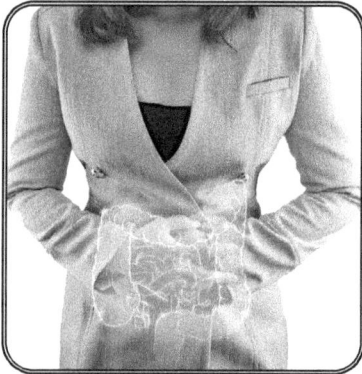

UNHAPPY BOWELS

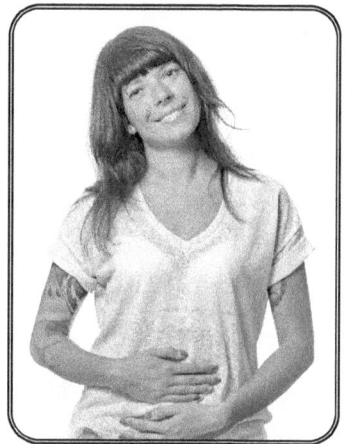

HAPPY BOWELS

5: Vitamins, Minerals and Other Supplements

5: Vitamins, Minerals and Other Supplements

No nutrition book would be complete without talking about these vital nutrients. I will mention each vitamin and mineral briefly because there are good resources that explain each nutrient in much more depth and detail.

Vitamins

These are micronutrients, as they are required in small amounts, but essential for numerous bodily functions. Vitamins are divided into two groups; fat-soluble vitamins and water-soluble vitamins. Vitamins A, D, E, F and K are fat-soluble, as they need adequate amounts of the correct fat and minerals in the diet for proper absorption. These fat-soluble vitamins are stored in the liver. The body excretes these via the large intestine as waste. Vitamins C, B, and P are water-soluble and cannot be stored in the body. These vitamins are absorbed from our intestines and bind to enzymes, and any excesses are excreted via the kidneys. The water-soluble vitamins are also essential to our enzyme activity.

No vitamin or mineral acts alone, so they need to interact with other vitamins and minerals before they can be utilised. Vitamin C isn't a cure for the common cold but is the principal nutrient in raising the body's resistance to cold and flu viruses. White blood cells can't absorb Vitamin C unless Vitamins B12 and B6, folic acid, choline and zinc are present in adequate amounts. This depends on the person eating nutritious foods and being able to digest and absorb them properly.

Vitamin A (Retinol) is a fat-soluble antioxidant nutrient that protects the body's cells against attack and builds up resistance to infection. It's essential to the health of the skin and mucous lining (the GI and respiratory tract) and for good night vision. Good sources of Vitamin A are animal products.

Another form called beta-carotene is found in red, yellow and orange fruit and vegetables. The liver will convert beta-carotene into Vitamin A.

The B vitamins
These are needed to release energy from our food and for the health of the nervous and digestive systems. These are water-soluble vitamins not stored by the body, so they must be obtained from our food daily. Generally, these vitamins are found in whole grains, nuts, seeds, beans, lentils, fruit and vegetables.

B1 (thiamine) enables the body to use carbohydrates as energy, which is needed for glucose metabolism and plays a crucial role in nerve, muscle and heart function. It helps protect against diabetic neuropathy and nerve degeneration caused by poorly controlled blood sugar.

B2 (riboflavin) helps to convert B6 into its active form in the body. A lack of this nutrient can hinder thyroid function and impair iron absorption. Enough B2 is vital for supporting one of the body's primary antioxidants.

B3 (niacin) is an essential serotonin component, helping reduce pain and induce sleep. It is good at controlling cholesterol and triglycerides, regulating blood levels of lipoprotein, and helping to prevent blood clots. It is also involved in joint repair.

B5 (pantothenic acid) is involved in many processes, like all vitamin Bs, and it's vital for the normal function of cells. It supports our adrenal glands in their manufacture of disease-reducing anti-inflammatory hormones. Our bodies use pantothenic acid to convert nutrients into energy and to make and break down fats.

B6 (pyridoxine) is involved in many chemical reactions in the body. It's needed to convert nutrients into energy, create our red blood cells, form our genetic material DNA and RNA, and break down an excess of homocysteine (amino acid). Like cholesterol, it can cause a higher risk of cardiovascular disease when present in high amounts. This vitamin is also essential for brain function, keeping the nervous system in good working order and supporting our brain's normal development during pregnancy and infancy.

Folic acid B9 deficiency is well known for causing congenital disabilities. It is needed for the health of the heart and the brain. It has been shown to have anti-inflammatory properties and hence pain-relieving abilities. Folic acid and B12 work together to create our genetic material, DNA, to form healthy red blood cells and support the normal functioning of our brain and nervous system. B9 works with vitamin B6; it helps to reduce and break down homocysteine, protecting against heart disease.

B12 (cobalamin) is needed in many important processes, like most B vitamins, especially for a healthy brain and nervous system. Vitamin B12 is obtained mainly from animal products. Involved in creating DNA and RNA, red blood cells and helping break down an excess of homocysteine.

Choline, phosphatidylcholine is a nerve builder and repairer; it feeds the nervous system. Eggs are the best food source of this nutrient, then greens, nuts and seeds. It helps the liver function. Choline isn't strictly a B vitamin; however, it is always grouped with B vitamins.

Inositol helps to reduce anxiety and stress, helping to relieve pain. Inositol isn't a B vitamin, although it is always grouped with the B vitamins. It plays a vital role in the structure of cell membranes. It also influences the action of insulin, a hormone essential for blood sugar control, and it affects chemical messengers in the brain, mainly serotonin and dopamine.

PABA (para-aminobenzoic acid), known as B10, is not seen as a true vitamin but is most often included in a B complex formula. PABA assists in producing folate in the body, although the amount produced is not enough for our daily needs. Best known for maintaining healthy skin, hair, collagen function and flexibility, and a healthy cell membrane. It has overall protective properties.

The B Vitamins appear together in food. However, most are lost in the processing of food, especially white rice and white flour. Those who drink or smoke, use the contraceptive pill or HRT (hormone replacement therapy), are under a lot of stress or rely on junk and processed foods, will have an increased need for all the B Vitamins. If you want to take any B Vitamins, always take a "B complex" unless otherwise prescribed by a practitioner. B Vitamins are found in whole grains, beans, lentils, eggs and green vegetables.

Vitamin C (ascorbic acid) is essential to the health of the skin, hair, gums, bones and ligaments. It is needed to repair and grow body tissue, maintain healthy blood vessels and red blood cells, fight free radicals, and keep the immune system in good order. It aids in the absorption of iron. It's a water-soluble vitamin that is not stored in the body. It's very unstable in fresh food and can easily be destroyed by oxygen, light and heat. Buy fresh fruit and vegetables, store them in the fridge and use them as soon as possible. Steam lightly or eat raw vegetables to preserve as much vitamin C as possible. We are one of only a few species that can't make vitamin C for themselves, so we need a good daily supply. A natural anti-inflammatory and anti-histamine, it aids the body's cleansing process and speeds up general healing. Coping with physical or emotional stress in part has to do with having enough vitamin C. During times of stress, including dealing with pain, the body uses up large amounts of Vitamin C. The adrenal glands produce the chemicals we need to deal with stress. Vitamin C assists in the manufacture of these stress hormones, and it protects the body from the toxins created by the breakdown of these hormones. Vitamin C is necessary for detoxifying. A shortage of vitamin C can weaken collagen, ligaments and muscles, and essential minerals are lost.

Vitamin D is called the "sunshine" vitamin, formed in the skin and activated by the sun. Vitamin D enables the body to utilise calcium and phosphorus, encouraging strong teeth and bones. Vitamin D can be stored in the body; if you take supplements, never take more than the recommended dose.

Vitamin E is a fat-soluble vitamin. It's a powerful antioxidant, protecting or delaying the onset of ageing-related diseases. Vitamin E helps maintain healthy circulation by keeping the blood vessel walls clear and robust. Nuts and seeds are good sources, although you should try not to eat roasted ones. Natural vitamin E supplements are labelled d-alpha-tocopherol, whereas synthetic vitamin E is labelled dl-alpha-tocopherol. The l has been added just after the d. In studies, the natural Vitamin E was found to be one-third more potent and twice as effective as the synthetic version.

Vitamin K is a fat-soluble vitamin essential to normal blood clotting and liver function. This isn't available as a supplement but can be found in some multivitamin/ mineral formulas. Dark green leafy vegetables, alfalfa sprouts and mustard greens are good sources.

Vitamin P is known as a bioflavonoid. This is a group of phytonutrients (plant compounds) found with Vitamin C in almost all fruit and vegetables. Each encourages the absorption of the other.

Vitamin U is found in cabbage. Scientists named this compound vitamin U as they discovered it helps heal digestive tract ulcers.

Minerals

Minerals are known as micronutrients or trace elements, performing many roles within the body. The body needs the following minerals - calcium, phosphate, potassium and magnesium - in larger quantities. Minerals required in smaller amounts are iron, zinc, chromium, manganese, copper, iodine, selenium, fluoride, molybdenum and cobalt. Minerals originate in the soil, are taken up by plants, and then utilised by us. The plants have converted them into a form that is bio-available to us. The same goes for farm animals that eat the plants, as they provide us with minerals in a form we can readily absorb.

Zinc, for instance; is needed to help make the correct levels of hydrochloric acid, which is vital for the accurate breakdown of compounds like calcium. A zinc shortage will hinder the proper functioning of our taste buds and smell receptors. This can encourage us to add too much salt to our food to compensate. This can cause further health problems as salt can inhibit our enzyme activity. Zinc assists many enzymes in metabolising carbohydrates. Zinc is needed to help fight infections and speed up wound healing. It also affects thyroid function, works with insulin, and helps to protect against heavy metal poisoning. Unfortunately, many minerals are lost in modern food processing and refining practices.

Boron is a trace mineral found in most plants. It's essential for healthy bones and muscles. Research shows that boron slows the loss of calcium and magnesium from the bones.

Calcium, as we all know, is needed for the bones, teeth, nerves, muscles and blood. Calcium promotes sleep, keeps the heart beating and the muscles contracting correctly. If you decide to take calcium, take it with other nutrients that aid its absorption. Good sources are yoghurt, almonds and sesame seeds. Dark-green leafy vegetables are how most animals get their calcium.

Chromium is a trace mineral involved in metabolism and, in particular, insulin production. Chromium lowers cholesterol and other fats in the blood. Molasses is a good source.

Copper is required in respiration to convert iron into haemoglobin.

Iodine is a trace element essential for the formation of thyroxin and tri-iodothyronine. An iodine deficiency can lead to an underachieving thyroid, with symptoms such as lack of energy, weight gain, dry skin, coldness, and slowing down of all body functions. Before you panic, some of the above symptoms could be related to other conditions, including stress, lack of sleep or other nutrients. Seaweeds are a good source of iodine.

Iron is a metal used by the body to make haemoglobin. This is the red pigment in blood. Haemoglobin carries oxygen to every part of the body. Good food sources are dark-green vegetables and meat, especially red meat.

Magnesium is a vital component of bones and teeth. It is closely involved in releasing energy and the correct functioning of the nerves and muscles. Epsom salts are magnesium sulphate; make a foot bath with Epsom salts and soak your feet. Your body will soak up some magnesium. Fish, beans, nuts, seeds and green vegetables are good food sources.

Manganese is essential to the function of the pituitary gland, the brain, nerve and muscle action throughout the body. It is vital to the body's antioxidant defence system. The body needs manganese to make interferon, a natural anti-viral agent. Oats, nuts, buckwheat, green tea, and whole grains are good food sources.

Molybdenum is essential for reproductive health; it helps the body detoxify, ridding itself of chemical additives. Whole grains, beans, lentils, leafy green vegetables and goat's yoghurt are good food sources.

Phosphorus is present in every cell in the body, and it's involved in most of the body's physiological and chemical reactions. It's needed for strong bones and teeth. This mineral is never taken as a supplement on its own.

Potassium controls the acid / alkaline balance, and it works with other nutrients to form essential electrically charged ions known as electrolytes that make up the fluids in the body. Potassium is crucial for many functions, including the heartbeat, energy production, nerve conduction, blood pressure and muscle contraction. It's found in fruit and vegetables; bananas and tomatoes are good sources.

Selenium is an important antioxidant that works in conjunction with vitamin E. Selenium boosts the immune system, keeps the liver healthy and combats the ageing process. Good food sources are found in fish, some nuts and whole grains.

Silicon (silica) is the most abundant element after oxygen. Chemical fertilisers and food processing tend to deplete it. Silicon is vital to connective tissue, bones, blood vessels and cartilage. It helps strengthen the skin, hair and nails by improving the production of collagen and keratin, the proteins found in the joints, hair and nails. Good food sources are oats, barley and brown rice.

Sulphur keeps skin and hair healthy. Rich sources are eggs, onions and garlic.

Vanadium is believed to inhibit the formation of cholesterol in the blood vessels; this mineral appears in tiny amounts in many foods. Black pepper, dill seeds, aniseed, celery seed and fenugreek seeds are good sources.

Zinc is present in every part of the body and has a wide range of functions. It helps heal and repair damaged tissue and is essential to many enzyme reactions. It is particularly important for a healthy skin and immune system. Zinc plays a crucial role in growth and cell division, which is required for protein and DNA synthesis. It is needed by the ovaries and particularly the testes to help maintain a healthy reproductive system. It is necessary for optimum liver function and for our ability to taste and smell. Zinc is involved in metabolising proteins, carbohydrates, lipids and energy. Seafood, whole grains and some nuts and seeds, especially pumpkin seeds, are useful sources.

> Vitamin C isn't a cure, but it raises the body's resistance to cold and flu viruses, and it helps faster recovery from illnesses!

6: AntiOxidants and Free Radicals

6: AntiOxidants and Free Radicals

Antioxidants are a class act. I find them fascinating. I am sure you have heard of antioxidants and free radicals. Free radicals attack us in a similar way that an iron gate could become rusty if not adequately protected. If you cut open an apple, you can see the cut surface go brown, and it's the oxygen that does this, which is free radical damage. Free radicals attack us daily, causing anything from wrinkles to cancer. Just as you paint your iron gate to protect it from rusting, we can protect and slow down the damage of free radicals by consuming antioxidants such as zinc, selenium and vitamins C, E, and A. There are also phytonutrients or phytochemicals known as plant compounds, and these antioxidants work in a similar protective way.

Some of the worst causes of free radical damage are smoking, too much exposure to UV from the sun, damaged fats (more on this subject later) and pollutants like exhaust fumes. Nature has provided foods rich in antioxidants, enzymes and coenzymes, namely fresh fruit and vegetables.

Here is a very small list taken from the hundreds of plant compounds with powerful anti-oxidant healing, protective and detoxification properties. They are anti-inflammatory and anti-cancerous, helping to lower blood pressure, prevent blood clots, strengthen the capillaries and much more. This subject is a book in itself.

Quercetin is one of the bioflavonoids with anti-inflammatory, antioxidant and anti-histamine properties. Quercetin may also help prevent or slow down nerve, eye and kidney damage for those with diabetes. Onions are a good source of quercetin.

Rutin is an antioxidative vitamin-like substance from the bioflavonoid group. Rutin supplements are used to treat capillary fragility and bruising, typical of many people with high blood pressure and bleeding gums. Buckwheat is a good source of rutin.

Ellagic acid is a phytochemical found in cherries, grapes and strawberries, and it protects against degenerative diseases.

Cruciferous indoles are found in vegetables like broccoli, cabbage, and Brussels sprouts; they protect against degenerative diseases.

Genistein is a phytochemical derived from soya beans (use only organic soy products as most soy is genetically modified). It is high in isoflavones, which normalises the activity of oestrogen and testosterone.

Glucarates are found in lemons, grapefruits and whole grains, improving detoxification.

Lignins are found in linseeds, carrots, beans, peas, whole grains and some fruits. They lower cholesterol and normalise the metabolism of oestrogen and testosterone.

Saponins are found in legumes (beans and lentils) and have protective anticancer properties.

Carotenoids are found in red, orange and yellow-coloured fruit and vegetables like apricots, pumpkins and carrots, and they help protect Vitamin A. Carotenoids help protect many vital organs.

Antioxidants have a vital role to play in the fight against toxic invasion and destruction. As we are all too aware, avoiding all pollutants and toxins is impossible. We can, however, endeavour to minimise the damage they cause us. Every one of our cells has its predetermined life span. Some live for hours, and others for days or months. Most cells can no longer reproduce correct copies of themselves after dividing about fifty times, so under normal circumstances, they self-destruct.

Our immune system becomes weaker as we age, making us more susceptible to infections. I know what you are thinking. We are often told that, according to statistics, we live longer these days, despite our Western diet and the toxic bombardment we face every day. However, in our not-too-distant history, the child mortality rate was very high due to malnourishment, poor hygiene, lack of medicine, lack of vaccines etc. This would significantly impact the average age calculation, thus bringing it down.

However, our goal here is to improve the quality of our lives, not just the quantity. As I said earlier, ageing is inevitable, but so much chronic suffering is not. Antioxidants help to protect us from ageing quite so fast, helping us reduce the onslaught of chronic disease and delaying or minimising the effect.

Antioxidants play a significant role in arming us with a powerful weapon against free-radical attacks. They are unstable atoms that contain an unpaired electron. Many years ago, I saw a book that showed these free radicals as bachelors at a dance that also showed happy couples dancing together. Along comes a bachelor who breaks up the happy dancing couple, leaving an unpaired free radical that was once part of a happy couple looking to break up another couple. They constantly search for other atoms or molecules to bind to and stabilise themselves. This can cause damage to human cells in many ways.

So, in practical terms, where do these free radicals come from? They come from both our internal and external environments. Internally, the body's many everyday metabolic processes produce free radicals as a normal by-product. Smoking, drinking alcohol, pollutants, UV, sugary food, processed foods and chemicals can cause free-radical damage that comes from our external world.

**Free Radicals
are seriously destructive
in your body!
Choose nutrient-rich,
antioxidant foods
for a longer, happier life.**

7: Toxins

7: Toxins

Toxins are a fact of life, and we can't escape them all. Toxins can come from our external world and are produced in our internal environment.

External toxins include heavy metals such as aluminium, arsenic, cadmium, lead, mercury and nickel. These metals can impair the function of the kidneys, the immune system, the liver and the brain. There are airborne toxins that come from car emissions, factory chimneys, glues and other volatile compounds found in new furniture, carpets, etc. Then there are preservatives, artificial sweeteners, colourings, food additives and pesticides. The most overlooked by most people are the chemicals from cosmetics, toiletries, pharmaceutical drugs, synthetic vitamins and minerals.

Internal toxins are produced all the time; they are the typical by-products of our metabolic processes and must be dealt with, regardless of their origin. This process puts a heavy demand on our organs of elimination, like the liver, kidneys, bowels, skin and lungs. Most of us make this process difficult for these organs, hindering their process instead of aiding and abetting them.

Is Your Body Struggling?

Signs of struggle are fatigue, sluggishness, being a little irritable or headaches, general aches and pains, and frequent infections of one type or another. We are led to believe this is normal and probably due to stress. Stress has a part to play, but we can't blame everything on stress. Stress encourages the body to produce certain hormones that are toxic long-term if the stress is not dealt with effectively. If you have any of these symptoms mentioned, it might be time to take a long hard look at your lifestyle (diet and habits) before things get out of hand.

We all lead stressful and busy lives with our work, families and financial pressures, and around all of that, we try to fit in the gym and have a social life. Then, to add insult to injury, we add more stress to our bodies through the food and drink we consume. Even the way we eat and drink adds stress. We are not giving our bodies the best tools and materials to enable the organs to function at their best.

Five principal organs of elimination work together constantly to break down destructive compounds into less harmful ones and allow waste to be safely excreted from the body, helping maintain an equilibrium. We have choices, though, to overwhelm or benefit these hard-working organs.

The **liver** is a prime example. It produces many alkaline-forming enzymes, which help break down alcohol, food additives, preservatives, water pollutants, pesticides and pharmaceutical drugs into less harmful substances ready for disposal.

The **lungs** help the body rid itself of carbon dioxide and maintain the blood's acid / alkaline balance – and a lot more besides.

The **skin** is a huge detoxifying organ. The skin excretes an enormous amount of toxic waste daily, especially in the summer when the pores remain open. In the winter, saunas and steam baths will open up the pores and encourage cleansing.

The **kidneys** are situated on either side of the spine, above the waist. These organs filter 900 litres of blood a day. They balance nutrients and fluid levels, excrete excess sodium, water and end-products of metabolism, including heavy metals, and the products of protein breakdown, which are ammonia and uric acid. When we use fat instead of carbohydrates, as in a "high-protein diet", ketones are produced and the kidneys have to remove them, which is a lot of extra work.

The **large intestine** is also known as our **bowel**. You should see a naturopath or doctor if you have had persistent diarrhoea. If the transition time is too fast, you may not have time to absorb enough nutrients and fluids, leading to malnutrition and dehydration. However, for most people, bouts of constipation are more common. Plenty of vegetables and fruit are needed, plus some whole foods, grains and pulses, as they all provide fluids, fibre and cleansing enzymes and nutrients.

Start by removing processed foods, and look carefully at the ingredients list! They say if you can't pronounce or spell the word, then absolutely don't eat it. Removing all those artificial substances from your diet is an important first step in reducing the toxins your body has to break down daily. Then there are all the creams and potions you put on your body and inhale from aerosols like hair spray. When I mentioned this to clients, many were surprised. Then I explain how nicotine, pain killers or HRT (Hormone

Replacement Therapy) patches work, e.g., through the skin. The penny drops about the creams and lotions. So, stop adding toxic substances to the skin and replace all your skincare products with natural ones that are so easy to find nowadays.

What to Avoid Putting on Your Skin

Aluminium is found in most deodorants. Aluminium is a known neurotoxin that can also damage the heart and lungs, cause fertility problems, and it has been linked to Alzheimer's. Found in deodorants and antiperspirants.

Coal tar is found in soaps and other products. It's a common synthetic colour pigment. It can contain heavy metals and can encourage the skin to become sensitive.

Formaldehyde can be found in nail polish, soap, shampoo and many more products. It's also the chemical they use to preserve dead bodies.

Dmdm hydantoin and **urea imidazolidinyl** – are two that release formaldehyde into the body, triggering skin problems, joint problems, dizziness and a lowering of immunity.

Isopropyl alcohol SD-40 is a drying and irritating solvent which disrupts the skin's mantle (protective barrier), making the skin more susceptible to other chemicals.

Parabens are common synthetic preservatives that extend the shelf-life of products, and these are found in many preparations. It has been documented that the chemical preservatives called parabens a) methyl, b) propyl, c) butyl and d) ethyl (alkyl-p-hydroxybenzoate) can mimic your body's hormones, becoming endocrine disruptors.

Phthalates are considered dangerous; they are found in many hair sprays, deodorants, nail polishes, perfumes, skincare and more. They can damage the liver, kidneys, lungs and reproductive system.

Talc is a mineral produced by mining talc rocks that are crushed, dried and milled. Processing eliminates some trace minerals but does not separate minute fibres, similar to asbestos! Talc is found in various consumer products ranging from pesticides to antacids.

Lanolin, Anhydrous (Ovis aries), also known as wool fat or wool wax from sheep's oil glands, is used in many cosmetic skincare products. It can cause allergic reactions and skin rashes.

SLS (sodium lauryl sulphate) Is a cheap detergent in typical commercial body washes, shampoos, toothpastes, exfoliants, moisturisers and shaving creams. It makes these products foam, and it disperses grease. In cream, SLS helps it spread further, which is known to damage the skin's protective outer layer.

Mineral oil is also known as white, baby, and petroleum oil. It is cheap and has an indefinite shelf life, so it is used in many personal care products. A petroleum by-product is not particularly beneficial for any skin type.

The same goes for the cleaning products you use, so replace them with natural cleaning products which are easy to find in the supermarket. One of the most significant home air pollutants is all those air fresheners!! They are huge sellers. Remove these chemical fresheners and replace them with 100% pure natural essential oils.

8: Water

8: Water

As we all know, we are just a big bag of water. All the chemical reactions needed to produce the heat and energy that enable us to think, feel, emote, express, see, hear and move, all occur in this fluid. Water doesn't need explaining, nor do I need to tell you how important it is, but research reveals that many people are dehydrated, causing long-term health problems. Being dehydrated is more serious and more common than you might think.

Water is our second most important nutrient after oxygen. Our brains are made up of nearly eighty-five per cent water and about fifteen per cent solid tissue. Our muscles are made up of about seventy per cent water. Many people, including children, are drinking themselves into dehydration by consuming too little water and too many beverages called diuretics that rob the body of fluids. Many people probably only get about a third of the valuable hydration benefits they need.

Water is vital in nearly every function of the body. It's a major blood component containing dissolved oxygen that is easily assimilated into the body. It helps prevent constipation, and the kidneys use it to flush out metabolic waste. Water helps maintain muscle tone because a dehydrated muscle is stiff and more likely to cause injury. Water acts like a natural "air conditioner", regulating our body temperature. It's crucial for metabolic reactions: when the body becomes dehydrated, the metabolism slows down, leading to a substantial decrease in energy.

As a general guideline, six to eight glasses are recommended daily because much will depend on your body size, your level of activity and the amount of dehydrating food and drink you consume, how much stress you have to cope with, and how hot the weather is.

Water is needed to break down protein, so if you increase your protein intake, your water consumption should also be increased. If you smoke or drink alcohol regularly, water is crucial for removing metabolic waste from the body. Water is the universal solvent, since it can dissolve and carry nearly any matter, including toxins. It's the indispensable inorganic element that dissolves, transports, lubricates, purifies, moistens and generally keeps us alive.

A serious concern is pollution from oestrogen and chemicals that mimic oestrogen. These come from birth control pills, hormone replacement therapy and other sources. Research by John Sumper, Professor of Biology at Brunel University, has studied the phenomenon of feminised male fish living in water that has been found to contain oestrogen substances. As oestrogen chemicals of various kinds accumulate in the environment, removing oestrogen from drinking water may be wiser than waiting for research to confirm the same fate for human males!

Water Filters

These are some of the most commonly used methods for improving the quality of our drinking water. The various methods of filtration and purification aim to remove three types of contamination:

Biological: bacteria, viruses, helminths (worms), and protozoa (parasites).

Chemical: pesticides, herbicides, solvents, chlorine, organochlorines, and hundreds of other chemicals.

Aesthetic: dust, silt, rust, sand etc.

Reverse osmosis is a technique of pumping water through a semi-permeable membrane. This synthetic membrane is a chemical compound which is relatively stable. Some RO units allow volatile organic chemicals to pass through. This is the reason some units include an activated carbon filter. RO also removes naturally occurring minerals, which has a softening effect on water.

Granulated activated carbon is found in the most widely used filters, including jugs, tap-mounted and most under-sink units. The main filtering effect is achieved by water passing slowly through the carbon granules, which have an enormous total surface area. This functions as an electrochemical absorbent sieve, removing contaminants like chlorine and improving taste and appearance. The carbon granules have been impregnated with silver to prevent the build-up of bacteria inside the cartridge.

Ceramic filtration is a technique that has been used for years. The effectiveness of ceramics depends on their pore size; the smallest goes down to one micron. Plenty of known chemicals and bacteria can pass through. This type of filter can be a good starting point for multi-stage filtration.

Multi-stage or combination filters use a combination of methods that can significantly improve drinking water quality. This is the sophisticated end of the filter market. Such a product can give up to ninety-three per cent removal of contaminants across a wide range of biological and chemical offenders. Naturally occurring minerals are not removed.

A **sub-micron matrix purifier** is an advanced system allowing filtration down to 0.1 microns. Particles within the matrix have positive and negative charges. Certain disease-causing bacteria are as small as 0.5 microns. This system doesn't remove naturally occurring minerals. Published research indicates 97 to 99.9 per cent purification throughout the life of each cartridge. Variations in design include under-sink, counter-top, portable or large-volume units.

Bottled water has several factors to consider: the cost, the amount of plastic or glass used in the manufacturing process, disposal or recycling of bottles and the overall environmental impact, including its transportation.

Club soda is artificially carbonated filtered water but contains added minerals and salts. The addition or removal of electrons has neutralised demineralised water, and the resulting water is called de-ionised or demineralised. This process removes nitrates, calcium and magnesium minerals, heavy metals cadmium, barium, lead and some forms of radium.

Mineral water is natural spring water, usually from Europe or Canada. To be considered mineral water, besides containing minerals, the water must flow freely from its source; it cannot be pumped or forced from the ground in any way and must be bottled at the source.

Natural spring water shows only that the mineral content has not been altered. It may even be possible that the water didn't come from a spring at all!

Springwater rises naturally to the earth's surface from underground reservoirs. The water is unprocessed, though flavour or carbonation may be added.

Sparkling water is water that has been carbonated. Naturally, sparkling water must get its carbonation from the same source as the water.

Carbonated natural water means the carbonation has come from a source other than the one that supplied the water. This does not mean the quality of this water is poor, as its mineral content is still the same as when it came out of the ground.

Steamed-distilled water means vaporising the water by boiling it. The steam rises, leaving behind bacteria, chemicals, minerals (like calcium, magnesium and potassium) and any pollutants. Once in the body, it is thought that the steam-distilled water will remove minerals and toxins the cells and tissues reject.

Smart Water is like distilled water as it is boiled, and the steam is collected like distilled water removing everything, including the minerals. However, the manufacturers then add calcium, magnesium and potassium.

Flavoured water has been sweetened with sugar or artificial sweeteners and contains natural or artificial flavourings. You will need to read the label carefully. You can make your own flavoured water cheaper and healthier by adding your choice of fruit, especially lemon juice.

Alkaline water has a higher pH level than ordinary tap water, as it contains oxidation-reduction additives. It is hard to find scientific evidence that this water will, as some people believe, neutralise the acid in the body. It is thought that it could reduce stomach acidity, lowering digestion and absorption efficiency.

Purified water has been treated to remove harmful substances like bacteria, fungi and parasites. This means that tap water is guaranteed to be safe to drink.

*****

We lose almost a litre (two pints) of fluid through our lungs and skin in breathing daily! Yes, our skin does breathe. Of course, this amount can rise if the weather is hot or if we work physically or train a lot.

Being slightly dehydrated can affect the pressure in the blood vessels; this can mean fewer nutrients like oxygen, vitamins, minerals and proteins are being forced into the cells. When the blood's osmotic pulling power is reduced, fewer nutrients get in, and fewer waste products are drawn out from the cells into the blood for elimination through the kidneys. Consequently, the more acidic the body's environment becomes.

The heart pumps about 130 litres of blood per hour. Amazing when you think about all that activity going on, unnoticed most of the time. A normal heartbeat is dependent on slightly alkaline blood. Acidic levels will eventually cause some level of deterioration in the heart tissue. If you have high blood pressure, consider drinking enough hydrating fluids and gaining enough fluids from foods like fruits and vegetables.

Drinking enough water also helps relieve pain and joint stiffness. If you suffer from headaches, maybe you are not drinking enough hydrating fluids and borderline dehydrated cells contract and retain waste. When you are well-hydrated, your cells expand, allowing them to eliminate waste products and maintain the correct pH balance.

9: Essential Amino Acids
(Protein)

9: Essential Amino Acids (Protein)

You may be one of many people just not getting enough amino acids (protein components) to control fluid retention, maintain muscles, aid healthy skin, encourage fat-burning, balance appetite, and so much more. On the other hand, some people consume far too much protein, which will also negatively affect long-term health.

Proteins are made up of amino acids. When we eat protein-rich foods, our digestive enzymes break down large protein molecules into smaller molecules called amino acids. There are twenty amino acids. Nine are called essential amino acids, as the body cannot produce these particular ones for itself. The other eleven are considered non-essential because our body can make them from other amino acids that we consume. We must obtain enough essential amino acids from our food daily.

Protein is Broken Down Into:
The nine essential amino acids:
Isoleucine
Leucine
Lysine
Valine
Methionine
Phenylalanine

9: Essential Amino Acids (Protein)

Threonine
Tryptophan
Histidine

Non-essential amino acids:
Alanine
Arginine
Asparagine
Aspartic acid
Carnitine
Cysteine (cystine)
Glutamic acid
Glutamine
Glycine
Proline
Serine
Tyrosine

Two from the above list are classed as semi-essential:

Cysteine

Tyrosine

Both these amino acids are synthesised in the body from methionine and phenylalanine. Even so, consuming cysteine and tyrosine regularly is a good idea so you do not use up your supply of the two essential amino acids, methionine and phenylalanine.

Each amino acid has a different effect on the health of the body in general. For instance:

Arginine, carnitine, phenylalanine, and tryptophan help to curb appetite.
Alanine helps with blood sugar levels.
Tryptophan calms the brain and aids sleep.

Isoleucine, leucine, valine, alanine and carnitine help build
  muscle tissue.

This is just a tiny sample of what amino acids do and how
important it is to consume enough daily.

Proteins (amino acids) are the building blocks of every
cell in our bodies. Muscles are the engine that turns the
food we eat into energy. Healthy muscles are crucial to
stability and balance, metabolism, weight loss and that
all-important weight maintenance.

Protein can be used more efficiently when we eat
enough essential fatty acids and complex carbohydrates. If
we don't consume enough energy, some amino acids will
be used for energy instead of rebuilding, repairing,
hormones, etc. If we have to use protein for energy, this
puts a strain on our systems.

We need protein for our brain cells, genes, and
hormones (like insulin, testosterone, oestrogen, thyroxine,
haemoglobin (red blood cells), immune system, and so
much more). Every second of the day, our bodies are being
broken and rebuilt, and ninety per cent of our body's cells
are replaced yearly!

In four weeks, we will have a new skin.
In twelve weeks, we have a new blood supply.
In twenty-four weeks, we have a new set of muscles.
Bones are constantly replacing. In about two years, we
  have a new vertebra!

The most wondrous thing about this is that you can produce
a new you, a better model than the one you have right now.
Making lifestyle changes will produce a superior result if
you incorporate the proper diet and lifestyle.

9: Essential Amino Acids (Protein)

Not Enough?

Why are people (mainly women) not eating enough protein? One of the reasons is that many women are addicted to refined carbohydrates and sugars, so by the time they have overindulged on refined carbohydrates or used up their calories on such food, there is little desire for protein foods. Protein foods are not addictive in the same way that carbs are. You can understand someone overeating with a whole packet of chocolate cookies, but would they eat a dozen boiled eggs? Probably not.

What is Enough Protein?

The general rule is your "palm size" for meat, poultry or fish. A chicken breast or leg is about the size of one's palm.

Protein foods are:
Natural yoghurt
Eggs
Fish
Shellfish
Cottage cheese
Chicken
Turkey
Lamb
Beef
Duck
Nuts
Seeds
Tofu
Beans or lentils + whole grains together

It has been estimated that the average woman needs approximately 48g of protein daily, and the average man needs about 60g daily. Interestingly far fewer men suffer from protein deficiency than women do. Here are some measurements to help you see what's practical:

Chicken breast 20g.
Piece of beef (size of your palm) 20g.
Two eggs about 12g.
Natural yoghurt 7g.
Tofu (3 ½ oz 100g) 8g.
Cottage cheese (1oz 28g) 7g.
Piece of fish (4oz 110g) 20g.
Natural yoghurt 7g.
Fish, such as salmon 20g.
Half a cup of cooked kidney beans 7g.
Half a cup of cooked long-grain brown rice 3g.
Half a cup of walnuts 4g.

Add to this large amounts of all fruits and vegetables. Eating lots of fruit and vegetables is important as they are alkaline-forming and counteract the acid-forming protein foods.

The old term "first class" protein referred to meat, poultry and fish, and this is now called "complete" protein as these provide all of the nine essential amino acids. A second-class or incomplete protein refers to beans, lentils or grains as they lack one or two essential amino acids.

If you are a Vegetarian or eat vegetarian meals sometimes, here is something you should know. Take a look at the following chart:

9: Essential Amino Acids (Protein)

Food	Lacks	Good Source
BEANS	METHIONINE	GRAINS, NUTS, SEEDS
GRAINS	LYSINE, THREONINE	BEANS AND LENTILS
NUTS, SEEDS	LYSINE	BEANS AND LENTILS
VEGETABLES	METHIONINE	GRAINS, NUTS, SEEDS
CORN	TRYPTOPHAN, LYSINE	BEANS AND LENTILS

The rule is simple – *remember to mix beans or lentils with grains.* In other words, always mix the first and last rows to ensure you get the amino acids you need.

For Example:
Hummus dip with rice biscuits.
Bean curry with brown rice.
Spelt bread and lentil pâté.

For the Average Vegetarian, Grams of Protein
Half a cup of cooked kidney beans 7g.
Half a cup of cooked long-grain brown rice 3g.
2oz (56g) goat cheese 14g.
Yoghurt 7g.
1 egg 6g.
A quarter cup of walnuts 4g.

Along with plenty of fruit and vegetables as these contain small amounts of amino acids.

For the Average Vegan (No Animal Foods are Eaten), Grams of Protein
Organic tofu (3 ½oz 100g) 8g.
Half a cup of walnuts or any nut 8g.

1 cup of cooked kidney beans 14g.
1 cup of cooked long-grain brown rice 6g.
Half cup flaxseeds 8g.

Plus, plenty of fruit and vegetables, which contain small amounts of amino acids.

Small amounts of amino acids are found in many foods that are not necessarily classified as protein/amino acid-rich foods.

Please do not get hung up on exact grams of protein. I have put down these figures only as examples to give you an idea. Do not weigh or measure anything, be relaxed about it. You know what a palm-size, half-cup, or full-cup looks like, so approximate is fine.

Then there is the important question, can you consume too much protein? The answer is yes... since high-protein diets can damage your health.

The Dangers of a High-Protein Diet

High acidic levels can increase the risk of gout, kidney disease or damage (this has been widely published), osteoporosis, colon cancer, heart disease and dehydration.

Too much protein leads to excess ammonia, causing damage to the tissue of the brain, kidneys and liver. Our organs must turn this excess ammonia into a less harmful substance called urea. Excess urea contributes to gout, kidney stones, arthritis and general tissue damage. Such a diet is also deficient in essential fatty acids (unless you eat a lot of wild game) and low in plant foods that are high in protective nutrients, fibre, antioxidants, enzymes and so on, which are the anti-ageing properties that we need for a long and healthy life.

9: Essential Amino Acids (Protein)

The Answer is Clear
We must look at the most traditional eating methods worldwide and how some of these societies still eat. Each time people move away from their traditional way of eating to venture into the cities for work and start to eat a modern type of diet, within a generation or two, they suffer all the things we do, such as obesity, diabetes, heart problems, arthritis etc.

In the past, diets consisted of the following:
Fresh fish or meat - in moderation.
Plenty of fruit – all sorts.
Plenty of vegetables – all kinds.
Water.
Natural yoghurt, sauerkraut, kimchi, kombucha, etc.
A variety of whole grains and beans.
Plenty of herbs and spices.
Seeds.
Nuts.
Cold-pressed oils.
A little honey or maple syrup occasionally.

Eating the foods listed above never made them overweight, but this changed in the land of plenty, where food is flown in from all around the world. So modern people have every kind of food to choose from, yet most overfeed themselves with calorie-rich, nutrient-poor foods. We have become malnourished in a land without shortages, rationing or crop failures, and our supermarket shelves are full.

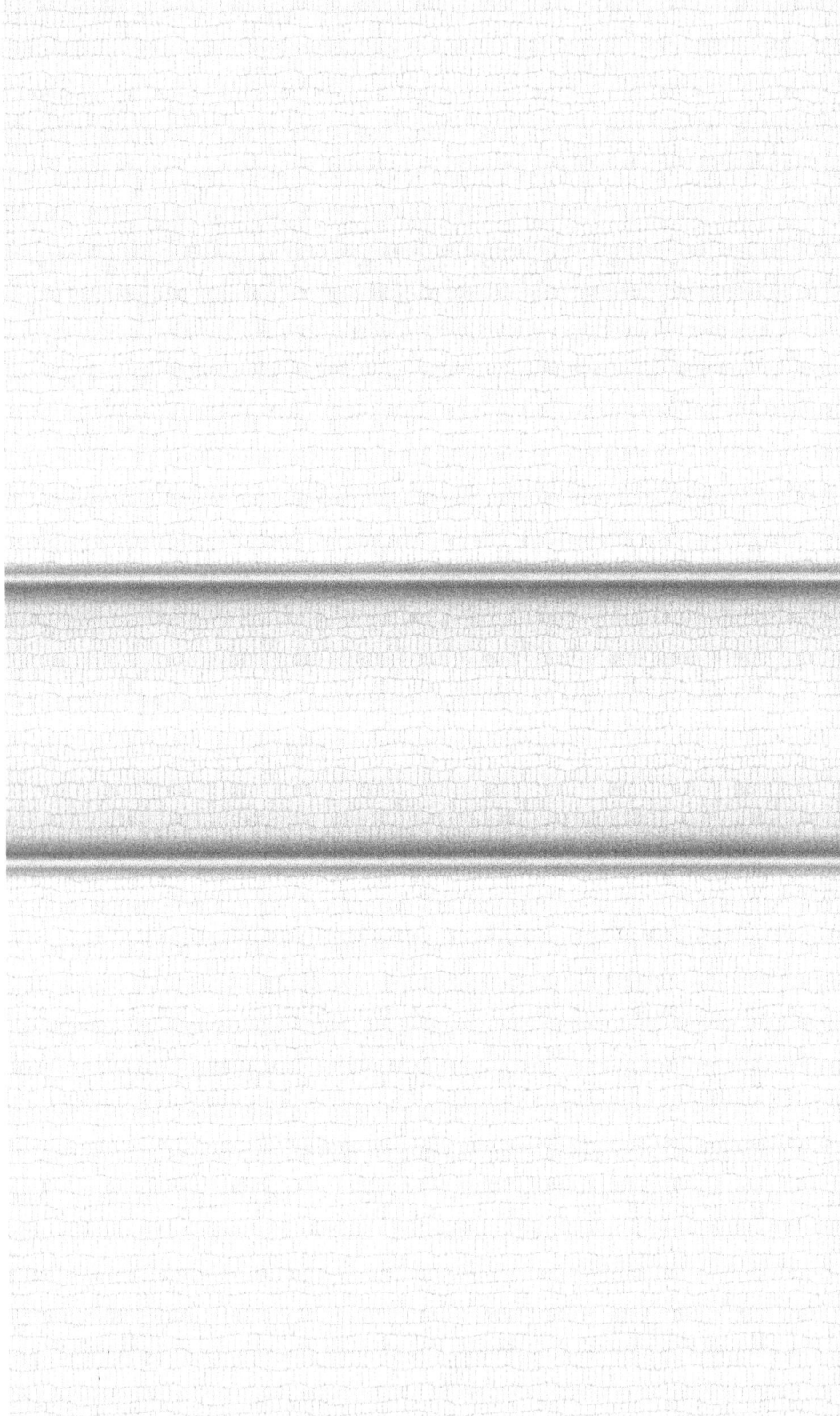

10: Fibre and Friendly Bacteria

10: Fibre and Friendly Bacteria

There is much more to fibre than you realise, but unfortunately, most people don't eat enough fibre from good quality whole plant sources.

Why Is Fibre So Important?
It helps you to feel full.

It helps maintain a balanced blood sugar level, preventing cravings and hypoglycaemia.

It helps to soften stools, helping to prevent constipation and piles (haemorrhoids).

Soluble fibre helps lower cholesterol.

It helps to speed up waste transition, drastically reducing constipation and auto-intoxication.

It helps to feed and encourage the correct bowel flora, the good bacteria.

It encourages the removal of excess oestrogen.

Getting plenty of fibre daily definitely does not mean eating bran! Bran is:
Not a whole food.

It is too concentrated.

It's too harsh for the bowel lining, often causing irritation.

It also lacks nutrients.

It can contribute to dehydration.

It hinders absorption of some vital minerals, especially iron and calcium.

It is better to eat food like brown rice with its fibre intact, unlike white rice with the fibre removed along with its nutrients.

Foods that are high in fibre, essential nutrients, plant compounds, and anti-oxidants are:
Beans.
Lentils.
Brown rice.
Quinoa.
Millet.
All Vegetables.
All Fruits.
All Seeds.
All Nuts.
Oats.
Spelt.
Buckwheat.
Linseeds.
Chia seeds.
Herbs.
Spices.

Our Gastrointestinal Tract is Outside of our Body!
You're probably wondering what on earth I mean by that. It is not until digested particles (molecules) pass through our gastrointestinal tract and move into the bloodstream that they reach our internal environment. In other words, inside the body. The gastrointestinal mucosa is a barrier between our external and internal worlds. This barrier needs to be kept healthy like any other organ in the body. It needs enough amino acids,

vitamins and minerals, enzymes, phytochemicals, friendly bacteria and so on or optimum function is impaired, which means it will no longer act as an efficient barrier/filter between the outside environment and our internal environment.

There is plenty of evidence to show that this can set up a problem known as a "leaky gut", and it can set up food intolerances, cravings and addictions. With the protective barrier compromised, larger molecules than normal pass into the bloodstream, setting up chain reactions within the body.

A healthy bowel is essential to every aspect of your long-term health.

Having a 'leaky gut' problem is an important issue in causing some health problems. This condition can contribute to problems like fatigue, headaches, cravings, bloating, puffiness and fluid retention, low blood sugar, skin problems, and more.

LEAKY GUT

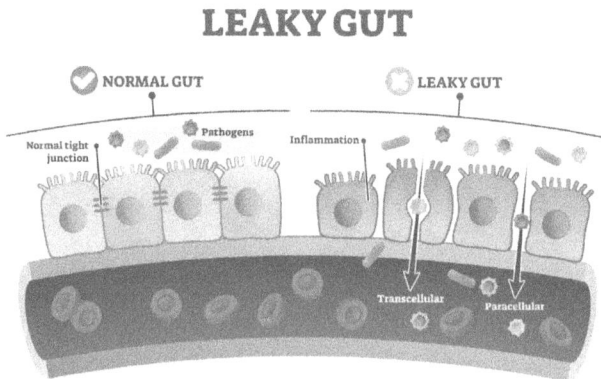

Leaky Gut
So how does a "leaky gut" come about in the first place?
From eating refined and processed foods and drinks.
Drinking alcohol (more than just moderate amounts).

10: Fibre and Friendly Bacteria

Using medication like antibiotics, steroids, HRT (hormone replacement), or contraceptives.

From nutritional deficiencies of one type or another.

From the wrong acid or alkaline environment.

Lack of enzymes, which is often due to nutritional deficiencies.

Lack of fibre, especially the correct fibre.

Bowel Flora

The average person carries about 3 lbs of living bacteria in their intestines, comprising an enormous variety and diversity of species. They have a direct or indirect, negative or positive reaction within the whole body, affecting every aspect of our health. The type of bacteria in the intestines has a huge controlling influence over absorption and general well-being. Much research has been done on how gut health affects brain function. The environment in the gut needs to be a little more acidic, and to achieve this, we need to cultivate the correct bacteria, known as "friendly bacteria". If the environment is too alkaline, the wrong bacteria thrive; the so-called "unfriendly bacteria" can flourish, encouraging auto-intoxication and inflammation. Auto-intoxication means your bloodstream absorbs toxins from your unfriendly bacteria, which burdens the cleansing abilities of the liver and other major organs. Friendly bacteria produce antibodies capable of rendering certain bacteria inactive, contributing to our overall health, reducing inflammation and even helping to produce some vitamins.

What Encourages the Unfriendly Bacteria to Thrive?

A diet with excesses of meat, wheat, sugar, milk, chocolate, tea and coffee, as well as smoking, too much alcohol, antibiotics or steroids, the contraceptive pill, and HRT (hormone replacement). Coupled with the lack of fresh foods such as fruit and vegetables, it encourages an environment that is too alkaline, which means that unfriendly bacteria thrive and take over.

What Encourages the Friendly Bacteria?

A diet rich in whole plant-based foods encourages friendly bacteria. This includes fresh fruits, vegetables, whole grains, beans and lentils, which help feed the correct bacteria. Plus, products that contain friendly bacteria like natural yoghurt, sauerkraut, kimchi, kombucha and others. These friendly bacteria help produce vitamins B and K and compounds that aid and protect our immune system, contributing to our health and helping every organ function more effectively.

Constipation

This is a common complaint, especially among women, and it worsens as people age. If you are constipated, you must prioritise this problem, as solving it will profoundly affect your overall health. Laxatives are not a good idea in the long run as they can cause potassium and fluid loss, leading to further dehydration. Many laxatives are irritating while they stimulate the nerves to encourage a bowel movement (peristalsis); eventually, a dependency develops due to muscle weakness, which ultimately contributes to worsening constipation, thus causing the very condition you are trying to solve. The longer waste matter stays in the bowels, the more poison it releases because fluids are reabsorbed into the bloodstream, giving the liver extra work. This is called auto-intoxication, and it contributes to chronic disease, poor skin, tiredness, weight gain, headaches, accelerated ageing, and more.

There used to be a saying that "an apple a day keeps the doctor away." The fibre in apples helps keep the bowels moving, so this old belief is still a good idea today.

11: Grains and Carbohydrates

11: Grains and Carbohydrates

Grains are grasses that produce edible seeds; some are kernels – they have four basic features in common. The outer husk or hull is generally not edible and is removed. Bran, rich in fibre, is the inner husk, the endosperm is the starchy centre, which is rich in carbohydrates, and the germ contains enzymes, minerals, vitamins and fatty acids.

What is Meant by Wholegrain?
These grains are as nature intended; the endosperm, fibre and germ are left intact, retaining the nutrients. Refining grains removes the fibre, the germ (fatty acid), and considerable amounts of enzymes, vitamins, and minerals.

Gluten is a sticky protein found in wheat, rye, barley and oats, and it isn't easy to digest. Wheat contains the most gluten – much more than the other grains, with rye next and oats containing the least. Gluten has unique elastic properties, much like chewing gum, which makes it ideal for making bread and pizza bases. This gluten can stretch to provide a honeycomb of cells capable of containing the gas produced by yeast as the bread rises. Until recently, barley bread was universal in the colder parts of Britain, but oats became more popular in the eighteenth century. Since the nineteenth century, wheat has been the most popular. Wheat is now overused, often eaten morning, noon and night, seven days a week, and many people only consume wheat or perhaps a little white rice, yet so many other grains could be included in our diets.

Phytic acid is found in high levels in wheat and in smaller quantities in soya beans. It can chelate (combine) with iron, zinc, calcium, magnesium, manganese, and several enzyme systems. It makes them biologically less available, setting up a chain reaction, depressing enzymes, and causing the pancreas more work to redress and balance.

Amaranth (gluten-free) is similar to Quinoa, a small round seed, pale in colour. It was discovered in Africa and Latin America and used by the ancient Aztecs as a valuable food. When amaranth is consumed, malnutrition is rare due to its high nutritional value and ability to thrive in very poor soil, even in drought situations. This poses the question, why isn't it grown more? Amaranth is a slightly more expensive seed/grain; however, it's a concentrated food high in protein and calcium. It's high in lysine, an amino acid low in wheat and most other grains. It contains more calcium and necessary nutrients like magnesium and silicon than milk. It's a rich source of fibre, easy and quick to cook, a good rice substitute, and the flour can be used to bake bread and cakes. It pops like popcorn, or it can be sprouted for salads. It has a mild, nutty flavour. Some health shops sell puffed amaranth as a breakfast cereal, with nothing added.

Barley (contains some gluten) looks a bit like brown rice. Whole barley contains more nutrients than the commonly used "pear"' variety, including more fibre, twice the calcium and three times the iron. The whole grain can be boiled in water, strained and drunk as tea. It's soothing to the digestive tract, helps stomach ulcers and lowers cholesterol. Barley can be used in soups and casseroles instead of rice or ground into flour for bread.

Buckwheat (gluten-free) has nothing to do with wheat. Buckwheat is a seed that is known as a grain. The whole grain has an odd shape, triangular with a light brown/pink colour. It's a good source of rutin, which strengthens the capillaries and blood vessels, reduces blood pressure and increases circulation to the hands and feet. It contains lysine, an essential amino acid not always present in some grains. Traditionally, buckwheat flour is used for making Brittany crepes. The whole grains can be boiled and used in salads or soups.

Buckwheat is commonly eaten in Russia and Eastern Europe, where it is known as kasha. There used to be a saying that echoed Napoleon Bonaparte's famous comment that "an army marches on its stomach" by saying, "the Russian army marches on kasha!" Kasha comes in various types, but the original pinky-brown type is the nicest, as it has a pleasant, slightly nutty taste.

Bulgur wheat (which contains gluten) is wheat that has been partially cooked, dried and cracked. Bulgur wheat is often used in Middle Eastern cooking, in dishes like tabouleh. Use amaranth, quinoa or millet as excellent nutritious substitutes to cut down on gluten.

Couscous (contains gluten) is made from granular semolina wheat. Again amaranth, millet or quinoa make excellent nutritious substitutes.

Corn (gluten-free) is also known as maize (corn on the cob). Native Americans traditionally cooked corn with lime. When other cultures started using corn as a staple in the nineteenth and twentieth centuries, it resulted in an often-fatal disease called pellagra, which caused wasting away. This was due to corn not having much niacin (B3). The old secret of adding lime increased the absorption of niacin. Eating corn isn't a problem for us as long as we eat a varied diet. Corn is a good tonic for the kidneys and the urinary system. This is especially true of the corn silk that can be infused and used as tea. Use the whole grain to make popcorn. Popcorn makers are cheap to buy and very easy to use, and children love them. As most corn is genetically modified, always use organic corn. Cornmeal is yellow, coarsely ground flour made from the whole grain; it is used for making polenta, and recipes can be found in most Italian cookbooks.

Kamut (containing some gluten) is an ancient form of durum-related wheat that flourished in Egypt over 5,000 years ago. Grown until the Second World War, when it became almost extinct in favour of the hybrid we know today. Fortunately, seeds were recovered from ancient burial crypts, and kamut is now being grown again. This is another grain that is well tolerated by those who have problems with conventional wheat or want to avoid overeating gluten. It makes a good substitute for wheat in bread making.

Millet (gluten-free), is a very small, round seed that is pale in colour and looks similar to quinoa and amaranth. It's known as "the queen of grains". Millet is alkaline-forming and anti-fungal, gluten-free and easily digested. It's a low-allergenic food and a good source of magnesium, potassium and Vitamin B3. Millet can be used instead of couscous, instead of breadcrumbs for stuffing, or in place of rice. The flakes can be used in muesli or to make porridge.

Hang a sprig of millet in your budgerigar's cage, and he will thank you!

Oats contain a little gluten, but much less than wheat, and they are one of the richest sources of silicon which helps to renew the bones and all connective tissue. Oats remove cholesterol from the digestive tract and arteries, and strengthen the cardiac muscles. It's a good source of calcium, magnesium, iron, phosphorus, manganese, Vitamin B5 and folic acid. The high fibre content has a mild laxative effect, making it excellent for indigestion, excess wind and an upset stomach. It's most conveniently taken in porridge, granola or muesli. Oats are used to make savoury oatcakes and flapjacks and are easily found in supermarkets. There is no need to buy expensive oats in fancy boxes because the inexpensive type in polythene bags actually tastes better!

Quinoa (gluten-free) is a cousin of amaranth and has some of the same outstanding qualities. It was one of the staples of the Incas and was called "the mother grain". Though not a true grain (it is a relative of the nettle), it is used as one. It has grown in the South American Andes for thousands of years and thrives in high cold altitudes. Quinoa contains more calcium than milk and is a good source of iron, phosphorus, B Vitamins and Vitamin E. It looks like millet, and it's hard to tell them apart, although quinoa is slightly darker. It has a mild taste and cooks like rice in about eight to ten minutes, which is quick.

Rice (gluten-free) is a staple for more than half the world's population. Jasmin rice, basmati rice for Indian dishes, arborio rice for risotto, black rice, red rice, short grain or long grain Patna rice are all lovely. Brown rice is a good source of magnesium, phosphorus, potassium, iron, manganese, Vitamins B3 and B6, folic acid and fibre, unlike white rice.

White rice has had the outer layer that lies directly beneath the hull removed during milling. The removed bit is rich in protein, fibre (soluble and insoluble) and minerals, Vitamin B and Vitamin E. This outer layer is used to produce vitamin-rich concentrates and rice oil. You would be much better off eating whole-grain rice than white rice. Brown rice flour can be used in various recipes, combined with other flours.

Rye (contains gluten) is a tough grain ideally suited to sourdough baking. It adds a slightly sour and naturally bitter taste, making it a valuable aid for the liver. This grain contains less gluten than wheat and is a good source of iron, magnesium, phosphorus, potassium, zinc, manganese and Vitamin E.

Spelt (contains some gluten) is a relative of wheat. It originated in Southeast Asia, was brought to the Middle East more than 5,000 years ago, and has since spread all over Europe. Spelt recently enjoyed a comeback in Europe because it makes excellent bread. Some people who have a problem with wheat find it easier to get on with spelt, in some cases, but it is not suitable for coeliacs. You can use spelt in any recipe that calls for whole wheat. Spelt is more nutritious, it grows a hard thick husk that protects the grain from pollutants and insects, and for this reason, it requires far fewer pesticides and other chemicals to keep it safe; this is good news for us and our environment.

Triticale (contains gluten) is a manufactured grain, a hybrid of wheat and rye. It's a rich source of lysine, an essential amino acid often missing in some grains.

Doesn't it make you wonder why the world is so full of wheat in the form of refined white flour products when there are so many grains to choose from that are so highly beneficial to our health?

Wholegrain is as nature intended: unrefined, with endosperm, fibre and germ left intact, retaining lots of enzymes, vitamins and minerals.

12: Seeds and Nuts

12: Seeds and Nuts

Most people would never consider eating seeds daily, yet they contain essential fatty acids vital to our health. They are also high in fibre. Add pumpkin seeds, linseeds, sunflower seeds and sesame seeds to your breakfast in muesli, yoghurt or porridge (after it is cooked).

Ideally, seeds should not be roasted. The food industry uses very high temperatures to such an extent the delicate and highly beneficial essential fatty acids in nuts and seeds are altered or destroyed by these high heat levels. This can turn a healthy fatty acid essential to well-being into a health hazard. This sounds dramatic but true.

To get the most health-giving properties from nuts and seeds, eat them raw as often as you can. The best-case scenario would be to buy nuts in their shells and crack them yourself. The shells keep the nuts and seeds fresh like nature intended, reducing the likelihood of damage from light and oxygen. Another benefit of shelling the nuts and seeds is that it slows down those who find it hard not to eat a bucket load once they get going!

However, buying shelled nuts and seeds is convenient, so ensure they have as long a shelf-life as possible and keep them in the fridge. Some recipes call for nuts or seeds, but home cooking uses lower temperatures than the food industry. Nevertheless, add them near the end of cooking to preserve as much of their goodness as possible. Occasionally, baking with seeds and nuts is all right, but eating most of your seeds and nuts raw is best.

Flaxseeds, or **Linseeds**, are very small, shiny, yellow or brown seeds. They are good at alleviating constipation and bloating, encouraging the elimination of toxic waste from the bowels, and helping to strengthen the blood. Flaxseeds are a rich land- and plant-based source of Omega-3 and Omega-6 essential fatty acids. Most rich sources of Omega-3 come from oily fish. Flaxseeds are also an excellent source of potassium, magnesium, calcium, iron, and vitamins B3 and E. These seeds are very soothing to the digestive tract due to their mucilaginous properties. They contain lignan, a compound that helps to protect against breast cancer.

Pumpkin seeds are green, flat and oval-shaped. They are excellent for the prostate gland's health and can help remove intestinal parasites. Pumpkin-seed oil is a rich source of essential fatty acids. They contain calcium, magnesium, zinc and B Vitamins.

Psyllium seeds are used as a laxative and intestinal cleanser. They relieve auto-toxaemia caused by constipation and bacterial/fungal infections. They contain calcium, magnesium, phosphorus, potassium and zinc.

Sesame seeds are tiny, pale-coloured seeds. They strengthen the heart, the cardiovascular system and the nervous system. They contain lignans, which act in a similar way to antioxidants. They help regulate cholesterol absorption from the diet. A rich source of calcium, iron, magnesium, zinc, Vitamin E, folic acid, potassium, copper, Omega-3 and six essential fatty acids. Tahini is made by grinding sesame seeds and sold in jars, like peanut butter. It's often used in dips like hummus (chickpea spread).

Nuts are a rich source of protein as well as essential fatty acids. The protein from nuts is easier to digest than that from meat. They are rich in linoleic acid, which benefits the heart and circulatory system. Like seeds, nuts should be eaten raw, but there are exceptions. For instance, cashews must be cooked due to a poisonous residue between nut and shell. The ones you buy in supermarkets have been cooked. You might see unsalted cashew nuts advertised, but chances are that they have been cooked twice, the first time without salt and the second time with salt.

Almonds grow mainly in the Mediterranean, but they are also cultivated in other parts of the world. If you cannot buy them with their shells, then make sure they still have their thick brown skin on them. Don't buy those that have been blanched (where a heat process has removed the skins). Almonds are a rich source of calcium, magnesium, zinc, some Vitamin Bs and E. They are also a good source of protein and are alkaline-forming. Almonds are one of the best nuts. It is said that they help regulate blood sugar.

Cashews are kidney-shaped nuts, originally from India but now cultivated in Africa and South America, and these are good for teeth and gums. They are high in calcium, magnesium, iron and zinc. They are only sold shelled (and cooked).

Coconuts grow on palm trees in tropical areas. The fat from coconuts is saturated (medium-chain fatty acid) but healthier than the saturated fat from animal products.

They also contain magnesium and potassium, and they can be good for   the thyroid.

Pine nuts are found in the Mediterranean on certain types of pine trees. Pine nuts are high in protein and essential fatty acids and are used in many vegetarian recipes. They are a rich source of magnesium, potassium, zinc and some B Vitamins.

Walnuts are native to the Far East. They are, however, grown in France, Spain, the USA and Italy. It is best to buy them in their shells as they stay fresh longer that way. They help digestion and improve metabolism. They are rich in calcium, iron, magnesium, zinc and Vitamin E.

There are plenty of other nuts to choose from, such as **Macadamias**, which are large nuts from Australia. **Brazil nuts** come from tropical rainforests and are a good source of selenium. **Pecan nuts** are grown in the USA and look similar to walnuts. **Pistachio nuts** are grown in the Near East and have a green colour.

All edible nuts have healthful properties, so add some to your daily diet, and some seeds for your essential fatty acids needs. They boost your protein intake if you are a Vegan or Vegetarian.

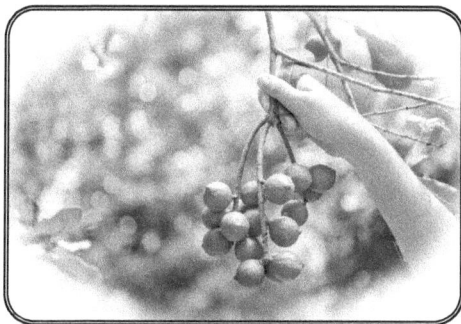

MACADAMIA NUTS

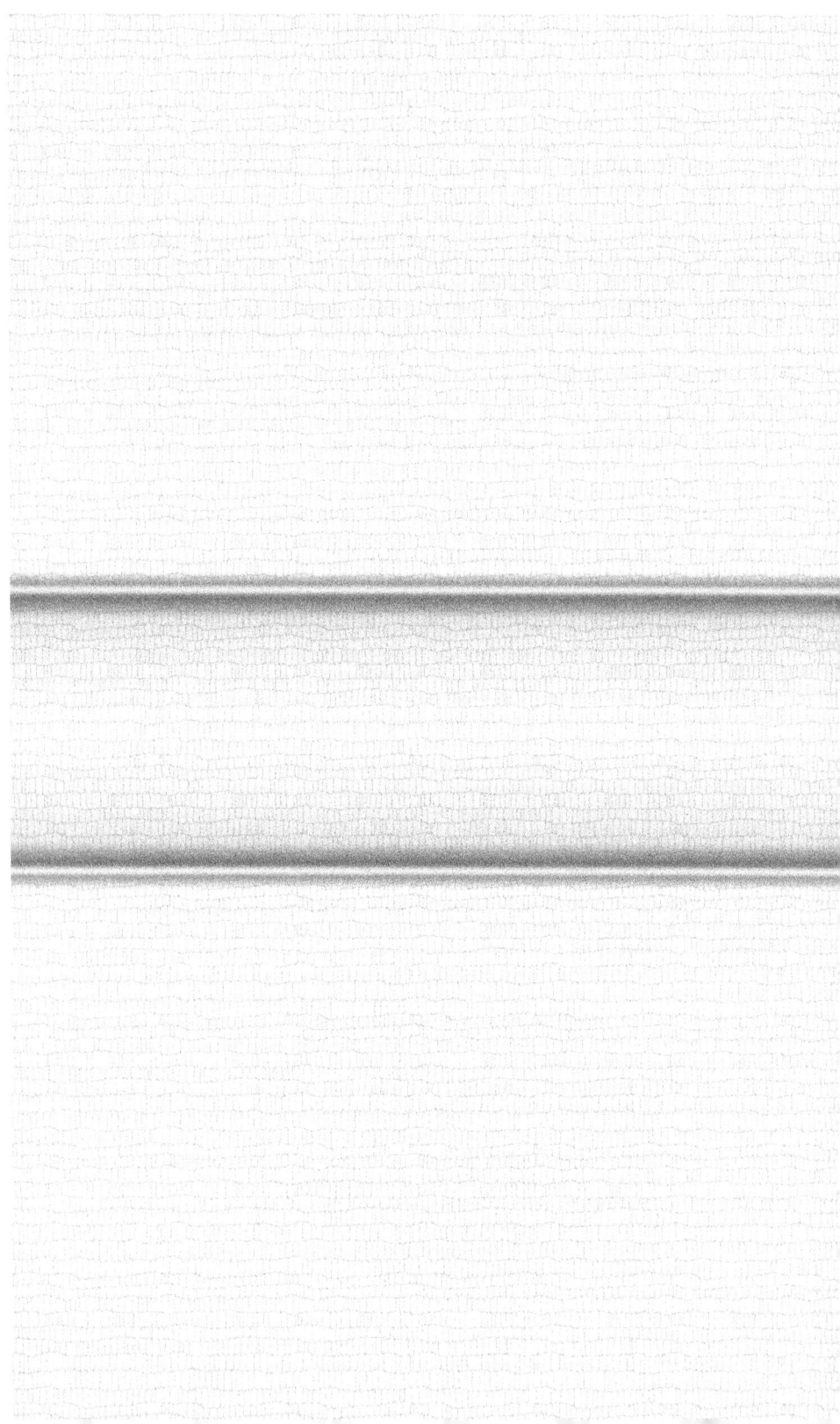

13: Beans and Lentils

13: Beans and Lentils

There are more than seventy varieties of legumes known as beans and lentils. They have been an important part of every known cuisine for thousands of years. In comparison to beans, grains are the new kids on the block.

Beans are high in fibre and low in fat and calories. Half a cup contains more than six grams of fibre plus potassium, zinc, iron and B vitamins. Beans are a good source of protein, although they lack some essential amino acids, but adding quinoa, millet, oats, barley or whole-grain rice to the meal will provide the essential amino acids that are missing.

Dried beans need to be soaked overnight, with one-part beans to four parts water. After soaking for at least eight hours, the water MUST be thrown away, as most of the gas-causing enzymes are released into the water. Then put the beans in plenty of fresh water and bring to the boil; while simmering, add salt or a little seaweed, cumin seeds, fennel seeds or caraway seeds to make the beans even easier to digest. They must be brought to the boil and then boiled rapidly for twenty minutes without the lid. After this, bring down the heat, cover the beans with a lid, and continue to simmer until soft. Cook large batches and store what you don't need immediately in the freezer for convenience.

Chickpeas are also known as garbanzo beans, and they support kidney function. They act as digestive cleansers and are a good source of calcium, magnesium, potassium, zinc, manganese, Vitamins B3, B5, B6 and Folic acid. Chickpeas are used a lot in Middle Eastern and Indian cooking. The flour from chickpeas is known as gram flour.

Kidney beans are high in fibre and they cleanse the digestive tract. They increase beneficial bacteria and remove excess cholesterol. They are a good source of calcium, magnesium, phosphorus, potassium and folic acid.

Lentils are a good source of soluble and insoluble fibre, along with minerals, for nearly every organ in the body. They neutralise acids produced in the muscles and provide calcium, magnesium and phosphorus. They are a rich source of potassium, zinc, folic acid and fibre. Lentils help lower cholesterol and are easier to digest than beans.

Mung beans are small, round, green, and they are a great heart and blood cleanser, excellent for detox. They are a good source of calcium, magnesium, iron, potassium, zinc, vitamins B3, B5 and folic acid. They are good eaten sprouted.

Peanuts, also known as groundnuts, are not nuts but legumes; they don't grow on trees or bushes like nuts. Peanuts are grown in the ground, hence their other name, groundnuts, and they grow in a pod. The Spanish stumbled across peanuts in South America, but China and India produce more than fifty per cent of the world's peanuts these days, and the US accounts for only five per cent. Peanuts can slow down the liver's metabolism and should be avoided if you are overweight. Peanuts are also heavily sprayed with agricultural chemicals.

Soya beans are very hard to digest, so they are traditionally eaten in a fermented form like tofu or soy sauce, tamari, tempeh, miso, etc. Do not overdo it; ensure that you only eat soy products in moderation and only eat organic products. Most of the world's soybeans have been genetically modified. Soybeans and soy products are rich in phytoestrogens, hormone-like substances that mimic the action of oestrogen in the body.

Tofu, also known as soybean curd, is part of Oriental cuisine and is a good protein source. It has only four to five per cent fat which is mainly unsaturated. The B vitamins and minerals remain undamaged by the tofu-making process. It comes in two types: silken tofu, which can replace cream in desserts and sauces, and firm tofu, which has a soft, cheese-like consistency. Tofu can be used in sweet and savoury dishes. Depending on how you view it, there is one drawback – or benefit – that tofu has no flavour at all. It's bland, but this isn't a problem as it soaks up any flavour readily and is ideal for marinating.

Tofu is made from dry soybeans, soaked and then crushed and boiled. A coagulant is added to this soy milk, separating it into curds and whey, a process similar to cheese-making. The curds are then poured into moulds and left to settle. It's naturally low in fat and calories. Only choose organic tofu and only eat it in moderation. Soy sauce is made from wheat, soybeans, water and sea salt. On the other hand, Tamari is a soy sauce made without wheat. Tempeh is also a soy product, made via an enzyme process that creates a white fibrous mass. Many varieties are made with a combination of soy, wheat, rice, peanuts or millet. High in protein and low in fat, do not eat tempeh raw as it needs to be well-cooked.

14: The Sugar Imposters

14: The Sugar Imposters

It has been estimated that more than 4,000 food and drink products are sweetened with artificial sweeteners. The Global Artificial Sweetener Market will be worth 9.6 billion dollars by 2026. Sweeteners have been a huge success in terms of profit for the pharmaceutical companies that produce them. You could be consuming much more than you realise, so read labels very carefully and look out for foods that contain the following:

Avoid anything that ends in "ose" - even when not actual artificial sweeteners – such as dextrose, fructose, glucose, lactose, maltose and sucrose.
Neotame.
Saccharin.
Acesulfame K, also known as acesulfame potassium.
Aspartame.
Alitame.
Cyclamate.
New ones are being invented all the time.

These Five are Considered the Worst
1   Aspartame.
2   Sucralose.
3   Acesulfame K.

4   Saccharin.

5   Xylitol (Erythritol, maltitol, mannitol, morbitol, sorbitol and other sugar alcohols that end in – itol).

All these sugars/sweeteners are available under many different commercial names, also differing from country to country. Look at the item's ingredient list when shopping.

Few studies have been done on the safety of mixing artificial sweeteners from various products or the long-term safety of artificial sweeteners combined with all the other food additives and chemicals consumed daily. So why would you want to consume something called "artificial"? Most dieters and even non-dieters use sweeteners or products containing them to avoid extra calories while still eating their favourite foods.

Many studies on both animals and humans have confirmed an ironic fact. Artificial sweeteners increase appetite and contribute to cravings for sweet and fatty foods! I doubt this is what you have in mind when choosing sweeteners. Studies have shown that a significantly higher percentage of users of artificial sweeteners gained weight than non-users! Animals fed these sweeteners become considerably fatter than those without artificial sweeteners. Some male subjects were given either artificial sweeteners or sugar, and both groups put on weight.

You may be surprised to hear artificial sweeteners can be very addictive, making it hard for some people to give them up. These sweeteners can become even more addictive when consumed with caffeine. Caffeine is found in cokes, coffee, tea, and even decaf contains some caffeine, as do some medications.

All of this puts considerable extra strain on the body's resources, using up reserves that would otherwise be put to better use. As you know, any chemical you consume must be broken down by the liver into smaller components by different processes before the body can render them harmless, as in the case of artificial sweeteners. They provide no nutrients but use up precious nutrients.

While some industry experts claim the molecule is similar to sugar, it is different. At the same time, other independent researchers say it has more in common with pesticides because the bonds holding the carbon and chlorine atoms together are more characteristic of a chlorocarbon than sugar, and most pesticides are chlorocarbons. The manufacturer's own short-term studies showed that sucralose caused shrunken thymus glands and enlarged livers and kidneys in rodents. But in this case, the FDA decided that these studies weren't based on human test subjects, so they were inconclusive! Observational evidence shows that there are side effects. Yet again, there will always be a sector of the population that is sensitive to something.

A note from Sasha, the editor of this book. Some people can't handle sugar, and they rely on sucralose for hot drinks and sweetening for home-cooked desserts. It may not be perfect, but for someone with diabetes, sucralose is a life-saver. I believe it is best to use natural products where possible, but if you have an intolerance to sugar, milk, gluten or whatever, and you have no option but to turn to some alternative product, you should do the best you can and not fret about it.

15: Sugar

15: Sugar

Sugar is seriously acid-forming, highly addictive and can effectively interfere with digestion. If you eat sugary foods, only do so occasionally, not during - or shortly after - a meal. Think for a moment about all the sugar you consume. Try to calculate the amount of sugar you are ingesting each week. It will surprise you; it's always more than you think. Read the ingredients listed on labels with great care. Sugar is so addictive that most people find it hard to give it up, and it is found in more products today than you realise.

Consuming sugar puts a strain on our immune system. It continually evokes an auto-immune response putting our whole system out of balance. Sugar enters the bloodstream too quickly, raising our blood sugar levels. This, in turn, triggers the pancreas to produce insulin, bringing the blood sugar levels down again. It does its job rather well and brings blood sugar levels down a little too much, thus causing a yo-yo effect and making most people reach for something that will raise their blood sugar levels again: something containing sugar or caffeine.

The liver converts sugar into triglycerides and then store them as fat. Many so-called "low-fat" or "no-fat" products contain sugar instead of fat to give flavour and texture to a product. These products will eventually turn to fat! Ironic, don't you think? Due to sugar's acidic nature, it can encourage osteoporosis because the body will draw on its calcium reserve to help neutralise the higher acid levels. The more sugar-filled foods you eat, the more addicted you become and the more accustomed you become to a sweet taste. The more acidic you become, the more inflammation your body will experience. Many people are totally reliant on sugar and stimulants like tea, coffee, cokes and chocolate to give them their oomph and help them cope with their day. They have become victims caught in a vicious circle that is difficult to escape. The more you rely on sugar and stimulants, the more tired you will become, and the more stimuli you use, the more deficient you will become.

Fructose in HFCS (High-Fructose Corn Syrup)
It is of great concern to me that people are confused between high-fructose corn syrup and the fructose in fresh fruit. Every week, someone tells me they don't eat much fresh fruit because they have read how bad fructose is. So now those who never did eat much fruit are eating even less or none at all.

High Fructose Corn Syrup (HFCS) is highly concentrated; it is made from corn syrup, and in the last twenty years, its usage has reached astonishing proportions. This syrup appears in a vast number of foods and drinks. It tastes like sugar, it is as sweet as sugar, but it's cheaper than sugar, which is why food manufacturers use it. Consumption of sodas (soft drinks) has skyrocketed over the last few years, and many are heavily laden with high-fructose corn syrup. HFCS is cheaper than sugar, but producers have another significant advantage; HFCS helps most baked products stay moist for longer, giving them a longer shelf-life for less cost. It's a win-win situation for them.

People have read that HFCS causes health problems and weight gain. They have also read that fresh fruit contains fructose, so they put two and two together and ended up with five. Don't make the same mistake of thinking that because it's called "high fructose corn syrup", you should stop eating fresh fruit and some vegetables because they happen to contain fructose. It's not concentrated, and it's not from genetically engineered corn. Fructose from fresh fruit is very diluted in its natural form by fibre and nutrients. It's not the same as HFCS.

Media headlines love to say misleading things such as, "One tablespoon of sugar has the same calories as a cup of blueberries". There is no need to worry about the small amount of naturally occurring fructose you will consume from eating whole fruits and vegetables. They contain the vitamins, minerals, enzymes, plant compounds, fluid and fibre needed for every aspect of good health.

Some natural sweeteners can be used as alternatives to white sugar, but they should still be used in moderation. It would be best to re-educate your taste buds to expect less sweet-tasting foods.

Dried fruit is a good substitute for sugar in recipes. Soak in water for a few hours first and then puree. Dried dates, apricots, raisins and figs are suitable for this.

Coconut sugar, more widely available these days, is less processed than white sugar, and like other unrefined sugars, it retains some of its natural vitamins, minerals, fibre and antioxidants. Remember, though, that by consuming this, you still maintain that sweet tooth, as it's a concentrated food.

Honey has been known for centuries for its healing properties. Cold-pressed honey is really the best, as the enzymes haven't been destroyed by high-temperature production methods that destroy enzymes. It has antibacterial properties, and it speeds up healing when used externally. Internally, it's soothing and calming to the intestinal tract and other mucus linings. It helps maintain electrolyte balance, especially during vomiting and diarrhoea. Buy the best quality raw honey you can find or afford. Be careful not to consume too much of it, though, as it will interfere with your blood sugar levels like any sugar does, so use it sparingly. Locally produced fresh honey can be used to help treat hay fever.

Muscovado sugar, or molasses sugar, is an unrefined, dark brown sugar that retains some nutrients and is not as sweet as other sugars.

Molasses syrup is thick and very dark brown. Two tablespoons contain almost as much calcium as a glass of milk, and it's also high in potassium and iron. Molasses is a by-product of the sugar refining industry. It's the syrup that remains after the sugar cane has been refined to produce white sugar. As we all know, white sugar is void of nutrients, so cooking and baking with molasses make for a healthier alternative. It also contains chromium, which is helpful for the health of the pancreas, enabling us to deal with sugar. It has quite a strong taste, and getting used to it could take some time.

Maple syrup comes from wild-growing maple trees and contains a few minerals. Use sparingly as it will still interfere with blood sugar levels like any sugar does. Make sure the maple syrup is 100% pure, as some types have been adulterated with cheap refined sugar or syrup.

Try to give up sugar-filled soft drinks and sweet stuff but keep eating fresh fruit for your health. Remember the old saying, "An apple a day keeps the doctor away".

Help with Sugar Addiction

Stop eating refined sugar and HFCS today; use honey, molasses and maple syrup instead.

Gradually reduce the amount of even these natural sweeteners, and your taste buds will begin to get used to less.

Begin to use dried fruit instead of natural sweeteners, then reduce the dried fruit and eat more fresh fruit.

You are gradually re-educating your taste buds to expect less sweetness.

For those using artificial sweeteners, start using Stevia (natural, no-calorie sweetener) immediately. Then gradually move to fresh and dried fruit.

Two supplements that will help with this addiction are:

L-glutamine.

Chromium.

Keeping your blood sugar levels balanced by eating regularly and not skipping meals is essential. If you maintain better blood sugar levels, you will begin to crave less sweetness while re-educating your taste buds.

16: Fat Phobia

16: Fat Phobia

Fat has caused much controversy and misunderstanding over the years, mainly due to the popular press. In modern society, we fall into two categories – one type overeating fat, especially the wrong sort of fats and those who try to avoid all fat at all costs, reaching for a "no-fat, fat reduced or low-fat or lite" list of products, perceiving all fats as the enemy. Not all fats are the enemy and some are vital to our health; these are called essential fatty acids. They are called essential for a good reason. We take these fatty acids in from our food daily, and they are essential for manufacturing a host of important hormones. Essential fatty acids are needed to produce all the prostaglandin hormone-type substances, which are ways the cells communicate with each other.

Steroid hormones are manufactured inside glands like the adrenals, ovaries, and testicles, whereas prostaglandins are produced in every cell of our bodies. All this depends on two essential fatty acids, linoleic acid and alpha-linolenic acid, and we manufacture Omega-3 from alpha-linolenic acid. However, a lot of people have become deficient in essential fatty acids. Most oils found on supermarket shelves have had alpha-linolenic acid removed. This enables the manufacturers to keep their oils on the shelves for months, even years, thus extending their shelf-life.

Our cells must be flexible and soft enough to allow substances to pass in and out, but firm enough to keep the fluid in between the cells out. At this point, we are literally what we eat. Essential fatty acids keep our cell membranes in good order and ensure they are flexible enough to allow the correct flow in and out of the cells. If we overeat damaged, processed fats, these produce harder and less flexible cells, making it more difficult for hormones, nutrients, and oxygen to travel in and out of the cells.

Facts on Fats

This is a vast subject, but I will tell you the story in a nutshell. Most of the information you have received over the years comes from advertising paid for by the oil and margarine industry itself. Advertising budgets can be substantial because this industry is worth billions, so why wouldn't they say their products are good for us? According to Dr Udo Erasmus, an internationally recognised authority on fats and oils, he discovered that some fats kill and some fats heal. Dr Udo Erasmus sifted through thousands of research papers before making his statement.

There are the good, the bad and the really ugly fats, which we know as "trans fats". Luckily after much pressure, the industry has been forced to reduce these destructive fats, but it took many years of pressure before the industry did something about it.

In years gone by, oil pressing was a cottage industry, and each large village or town would have a press. Once the oil was produced, it was handled carefully as light, oxygen and heat would easily damage its beneficial properties. The oils were bought in small quantities, stored in dark glass bottles, kept in a cool place, and had a reasonably short shelf life. As the industry grew, enormous continuous-feed, screw-type, heat-producing oil presses were built to replace the small, slow, cold-temperature presses. Automation made their operation highly efficient, which cut labour costs. Natural nutrients are removed from the oil, like carotene, vitamin E, and lecithin, making the oil "pure". These nutrients are potent antioxidants known to protect the heart. Some synthetic antioxidants (AOs) are added to refined oils as they extend the oil's shelf-life, but this is for the industry's benefit, not our health benefit.

Many things happen to nutritious seeds during their complicated journey to becoming colourless, tasteless oils that have been stripped of all their nutrients. The various processing stages create synthetic molecules our bodies cannot handle. These fats are toxic to the body and will add to cell rigidity, hindering the flow of nutrients and oxygen. These oils and fats certainly don't supply the body with the necessary raw materials to produce adequate hormones.

These oils also make margarine by another process called hydrogenation. The oil is put under pressure with hydrogen gas at high temperatures in the presence of a metal catalyst that is 50% nickel and 50% aluminium, further damaging the oil. The oils become "saturated" with hydrogen, making them solid at room temperature. These processed oils have been shown to increase cholesterol! They decrease beneficial high-density lipoprotein (HDL) and interfere with our liver's detoxification system.

The very word cholesterol instils fear, but you may or may not know that our liver produces about 70% of our cholesterol needs, and about 30% comes from our diets. Our bodies need cholesterol to produce oestrogen, testosterone, adrenaline, and D vitamins, to name but a few. If you avoid cholesterol foods altogether, the liver will have to create some for you. According to much research, these processed vegetable oils account for 74% of the plaque build-up in our arteries. Processed fats need to be metabolised like everything else we consume, creating an essential fatty acid shortage.

Extra Virgin olive oil is cold-pressed and does not undergo numerous processing stages. It contains Omega-9, and it is also known as mono-unsaturated. Research shows that this oil protects against cardiovascular disease. It positively affects the brain, is associated with lower incidences of cancer, and contributes to general good health. Other cold-pressed oils can be found in health shops and some supermarkets.

Look out for these terms:
  First pressed.
  Extra virgin.
  Cold pressed.
  Expelled.

Eating refined, processed oils, margarine and shortenings causes an imbalance in the type of prostaglandins we produce. Two classes of essential fatty acids are needed in our diet, and these are Omega-3 and Omega-6. Omega 6 is converted into three types of hormone-like substances. One type has an anti-inflammatory effect called series-1 prostaglandin. The second type, series-2 prostaglandins, involves inflammation and thickening of the blood. The third type is series-3 prostaglandins; they have an anti-inflammatory effect. These three need to be in balance. These days, the balance is tipped in favour of inflammation.

Nutrition in Focus

We are Eating too Much:
Processed oil and fat.
Too much saturated animal fat.
Too much sugar (turns to fat and triglycerides).

We are Eating too Little
Fish (especially oily fish).
Wild game.
Raw nuts and seeds.
Plants, like avocado.

If you don't eat fish or wild game, which provide EPA (eicosapentaenoic acid), you have a mechanism in place to convert alpha-linolenic acid into EPA. Sounds good in theory. It relies on enough nutrients like vitamin B6, vitamin C, magnesium and zinc to enable the body to convert alpha-linolenic acid to EPA. Most people on an average diet do not get enough of these nutrients. Excess consumption of processed oils can also block the conversion.

Foods rich in B6, Vitamin C, magnesium and zinc are fruit, vegetables, nuts, seeds, legumes and whole grains.

Inflammatory conditions are common these days because our diets block our natural pathways for producing the correct amounts of series-1 and series-3 prostaglandins that help balance inflammatory processes.

DHA (docosahexaenoic acid)

As we age, our bodies release chemicals known as cytokines, which encourage degeneration, inflammation and pain. Research has revealed that taking DHA (docosahexaenoic acid) found in fish oil can suppress the release of these cytokines. DHA is an Omega-3 essential fatty acid.

Flaxseeds, Also Known as Linseeds
These seeds contain about 40% alpha-linolenic acid. This oil gives us more flexibility than any other oil derived from seeds or nuts. Walnuts are useful, but they only contain about 10% alpha-linolenic acid. Most people think of linseed oil as a preservative for wood, and the linseed oil sold in do-it-yourself shops is not for human consumption. It gives life to dull wood and helps to preserve it – but much in the same way, edible linseed will give life to the body and help to preserve it. It provides flexibility to cells, enabling them to function better and allowing for better communication between the cells by producing prostaglandins while encouraging a reduction in inflammation.

From Sugar to Triglyceride Fat
Sugar is broken down into smaller molecules, eventually ending up as triglycerides, which are fats in the blood. What are the implications of higher levels of triglycerides? Impaired blood flow, higher risk of narrowing arteries and raised insulin levels, which raise triglyceride and cholesterol levels.

> **Extra Virgin and other cold-pressed oils help to protect against cardiovascular disease. The other processed oils account for 74% of plaque build-up in our arteries.**

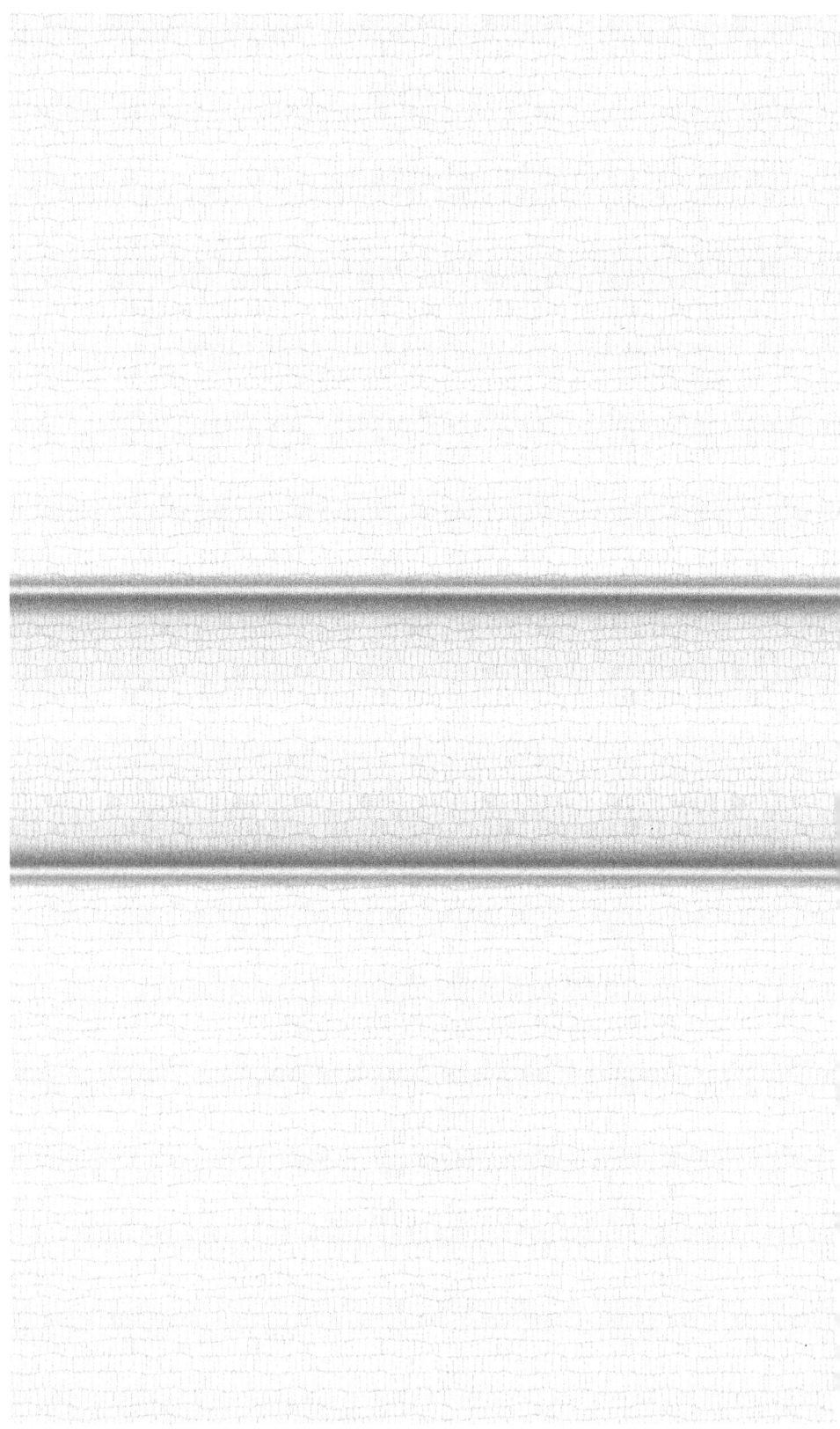

17: Hormones and Nutrition

17: Hormones and Nutrition

On hearing the word insulin, most people think of diabetes, but there is much more to insulin. Western diets produce too much insulin, our cells become bombarded and overwhelmed, and they stop responding as efficiently as they should. This developing sensitivity to insulin at a cellular level contributes to various conditions, such as inflammation and pain, heart disease, obesity, tiredness, diabetes and arteriosclerosis.

Too Much Insulin
Eating refined carbohydrates and sugars, we cause a sudden rise in our blood sugar levels because large amounts enter the bloodstream too quickly, which triggers insulin production. Triglyceride levels increase (fats from sugar), and high-density levels increase (known as "bad" guys), eventually causing insulin resistance because the cells stop responding as effectively as they should. Over the years, this can destroy insulin-secreting beta-cells in the pancreas, not due to your chronological age but to your lifestyle.

Five Inflammatory Substances
Histamine – the mast cells produce histamine. I am sure you have heard of anti-histamine medication. Histamine

is involved in the immune process. For example, asthma, eczema and hay fever sufferers produce high histamine levels.

To Counteract Histamine, Eat:
Fruits such as blackcurrants, kiwis and cherries.
Vegetables such as onions and garlic.
Supplements, such as vitamin C and quercetin.
L-methionine capsules help the liver detox and bind to excess histamine, rendering it inactive.

Kinins – found circulating in the bloodstream, they're produced in response to tissue damage caused by the following:
High acidity levels.
Stress.
High protein diets.
Dehydration.
Certain foods and drinks.

To counteract kinins, you need a diet high in fruit and vegetables (and other foods in moderation). This will reduce acidity and maintain a good balance between acid and alkaline.

Prostaglandins – which are short-lived hormone-type substances. They affect tissue in their immediate area. The prostaglandins produced are called 1, 2, or 3, directly resulting from the foods we eat. Prostaglandins 1 and 3 are very important as anti-inflammatory substances and help reduce cholesterol, prevent blood clots, and maintain good blood pressure. To maintain good balance, eat the following:

Fresh fruit and vegetables.

Ginger.

Vitamin C.

B Complex.

Minerals like magnesium and zinc are vital for enzyme production that quell pro-inflammation.

Flaxseed oil capsules or fish oil.

A diet that provides enough essential fatty acids like fish, raw nuts and seeds.

Leukotrienes – little is known about these substances. They are related to prostaglandins and are generated from arachidonic acid, which comes from a diet high in animal products. To counter leukotrienes, eat the following:

Vegetables, such as onions.

Spice, such as turmeric.

Quercetin capsules.

L-Arginine capsules.

Turmeric capsules.

Complement. You may not have heard of this. It is a protein found in the bloodstream, and about a dozen different substances work with the immune system. In other words, these substances complement the immune system. They dilate arterioles, tiny arteries that feed the tiny blood capillaries. This is also involved in the release of histamine from the mast cells encouraging inflammation. Various nutrients and antioxidants are needed as follows:

Vitamin A or beta-carotene.

Vitamin C.

Vitamin E.

Selenium.

Zinc.

Fruits and vegetables that are coloured red, yellow and orange, like pumpkin, beetroot, squash, carrots, berries, nectarines, etc.

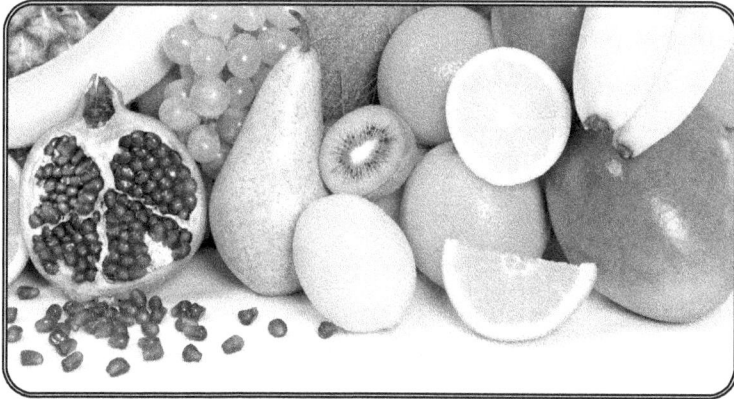

FRESH FRUIT

18: Five a Day

18: Five a Day

This refers to the amount of fruit and vegetables we should eat daily, and it is the very minimum daily requirement given to the general public as a guideline. Evidence shows few people consume that much fresh plant-based food in a week, let alone a day, unless you count tomato ketchup and potatoes! For all the campaigning, the message just isn't getting through, or perhaps people don't believe it will make much difference to them.

It is imperative to our overall health that we consume fresh fruit and vegetables daily and that we choose more than five a day for nourishment, detoxing and repair. More than five portions a day will maintain the correct pH balance to regenerate healthy cells, protect from cancer, help maintain hormone balance, guard against inflammation, and so much more.

More Fruit
Put out a well-stocked fruit bowl somewhere easily seen and reached by all family members. For some people, if it's out of sight, it's out of mind. Peel fruit for children and keep it in a container in the fridge. Given the opportunity, children will eat fruit if you have prepared it for them, and this also goes for some adults! I know people who won't eat fruit from

a fruit bowl but are more than happy to eat a prepared fruit salad. Also, make your own smoothies.

More Vegetables
   Vegetable soups.
   Stir-fries.
   Salads.
   Steamed.
   Stews and casseroles.
   In smoothies with some fruit.
   Cut raw vegetables into sticks for dips.
   Cut into thin spirals to use instead of pasta.

Fresh fruit and vegetables are essential in our quest to turn our degeneration into regeneration. They are so easy to come by, and they are available just about everywhere.

Buying plenty of fresh produce need not be expensive, and for those on a tight budget, there are always locally-grown seasonal fruit and vegetables. They are far less costly than imported produce out of season, but you could also consider growing your own fruit and vegetables. Maybe you can find small producers or enthusiastic gardeners who grow too much for their own needs and sell off the excess. Local farmer's markets or farm shops are also good places, as are pick-your-own fruit and vegetable farms. These all save you money. Some books show you how to grow fruit and veg in pots and boxes. Sounds a little crazy, but you can use carrot tops, celery bottoms, avocado stones, cabbage bottoms, and much more to regrow produce.

Of course, organically grown produce is better for your health and the environment. But if this is unavailable or beyond your budget, wash your fruit and vegetables well or peel them. At the very least, avoid genetically modified and irradiated fruit and vegetables.

Some people say that we should only eat organic vegetables and fruit or we shouldn't eat frozen or tinned goods, and in a perfect world, this would be ideal, but we don't live in a perfect world. Plenty of well-washed non-organic fruit and vegetables are better than processed foods or not eating as much because they are not organic. People often ask about frozen fruit and vegetables. These are good when you are in a hurry or have run out of fresh fruit and vegetables, and they can help if you are on a budget because they are often less expensive, and there is no waste. Tinned and frozen goods are always better than nothing or resorting to a refined, processed meal instead.

Fruits are cleansing and purging, whereas vegetables are restorative, so they are the perfect partners. They are alkalising and require little energy to digest, and it is impossible to embark on any health program without them.

Eating a lot of fruit and vegetables might seem a little overwhelming initially. You can start with a minimum of five a day and gradually increase your consumption over a period of time, eventually aiming for seven or more portions a day.

Buying Fruit and Vegetables
When fruit or vegetables are picked, they begin to lose some of their nutrients and enzymes, so try to buy sun-ripened, fresh-looking undamaged produce, as bruising and rough handling can destroy nutrients. Most supermarkets offer pre-washed, pre-cut vegetables, salads and fruit. The exposed cut surfaces lose nutrients very rapidly, and you pay a premium for them. Avoid buying your produce that way, except occasionally for convenience and speed or if you have arthritis and find it hard to peel and cut vegetables.

18: Five a Day

Store your fresh fruit and vegetables (except bananas or potatoes) in the refrigerator or a cool place away from sunlight.

Fruit and vegetables should be washed and cut just before eating or cooking. Never immerse or soak your fruit and vegetables for long. The peel is a good source of fibre and nutrients, so avoid peeling if possible.

Apples, cucumber and lemons are often sprayed or dipped into a heavy wax (you can feel it and see it if you look closely). This wax contains chemicals and would be better peeled, but it is best to buy unwaxed produce. You will find peeling and chopping vegetables quicker and easier if you have a good quality sharp knife, and it is well worth the investment. It will save you time in the long run. Chefs will tell you that you are more likely to cut yourself with a blunt knife.

I have a few gadgets that enable me to quickly cut vegetables into interesting shapes, but an electric food processor will grate, chop, or slice in seconds.

Boiling vegetables in water and throwing the water away means throwing away the water-soluble vitamins, such as vitamins C and B, plus selenium and potassium. If you boil your vegetables come what may, use the water. Either drink it or save it for stock, gravy or soup.

Avoid aluminium cookware as this can lodge in the brain and bring on early dementia.

Micro-waving changes the molecular structure of food. We don't know the effects of this change on our long-term health. I know some of you will continue to use your microwaves, but at least cut down the amount of microwaved food you eat and avoid microwaving your food in plastic containers.

Never deep-fry vegetables, as fat-soluble nutrients such as vitamins E and A are lost. Plus, high temperatures needed for deep-frying change the structure of the oil in an unhealthy way.

Salads

Make your salads more interesting than just lettuce, tomatoes and cucumber. Forget the iceberg variety of lettuce, as it's nutritionally poor and tasteless. Instead, use the following:

Chinese cabbage.
Chicory.
Rocket leaves.
Apples.
Pears.
Red lettuce.
Carrots.
Courgettes (zucchini).
Beans.
Fresh herbs.
Celery.
Spring onions.
Walnuts.
Avocado.
Red beetroot.
Peppers red and yellow.
Radishes (white and red).
Young fresh spinach.
Chives.
Mango.
Any type of sprouts.
Asparagus (steamed a little).
Artichokes.

Raw cauliflower.

Cabbage (red, white or green).

Fresh fennel bulb.

Any vegetable, such as green string beans, lightly steamed and cooled.

Salad Dressing

1 part cold-pressed olive oil.

1 part cold-pressed walnut oil.

Organic apple cider vinegar, to taste.

Freshly grated ginger.

Pepper.

Quality salt like Himalayan.

Or

1 part cold-pressed olive oil.

1 part cold-pressed hemp oil.

Fresh lemon juice, to taste.

Fresh chilli chopped small.

Freshly ground black pepper.

Quality salt like Himalayan.

Or

1 part cold-pressed olive oil.

1 part cold-pressed hemp oil.

Fresh lemon or apple cider vinegar.

Lots of fresh herbs chopped up.

Freshly ground black pepper.

Quality salts like Himalayan or Celtic salt.

Stir-Frying

Stir-frying is a quick, tasty and healthy way to eat more vegetables. A gadget that slices and chops vegetables thinly, quickly and easily would be good. This ideal meal is quick to prepare when you get home from work.

With some practice and the right equipment, stir-frying can quickly create various delicious meals. This technique evolved as a way of conserving fuel by cooking thinly sliced food quickly over high heat. Steel woks with high sides and rounded bottoms are inefficient when used on modern cooker tops as they cook too slowly and unevenly. The best type of wok is cast iron, which distributes and holds heat evenly throughout cooking.

Ingredients must be added to the pan in order of relative cooking time, with longer cooking items added first. All the ingredients must be prepared just before you start cooking. Uncooked seafood, fish, poultry and thinly sliced meat are stir-fried first and then removed while all the other ingredients are cooked, and then the meat is returned at the end. Use a teaspoon to a tablespoon of cold-pressed sesame oil or coconut oil. Do not overcook the vegetables because they should be just al-dente (just a little on the crunchy side).

Ingredients
Almost any vegetable can be stir-fried.
Some fruits like pineapple or mango.
Spices and herbs like - ginger, lemongrass or coriander.
Sprouts of any kind.
Chicken.
Meat.
Fish.
Seafood.
Organic tofu.

Lightly Steamed Vegetables
This is a healthy way of cooking vegetables as long as they are not overcooked. You can buy a multi-layered pot you

put on the cooker top or an electrical steamer. Most vegetables take about three to five minutes, although Brussel sprouts take about ten minutes.

Stews and casseroles are lovely with plenty of vegetables added – especially onions and carrots.

You can make endless soups with vegetables, beans, lentils, millet, quinoa or meat, but always add plenty of vegetables. Remember to add lots of onions, herbs or spices.

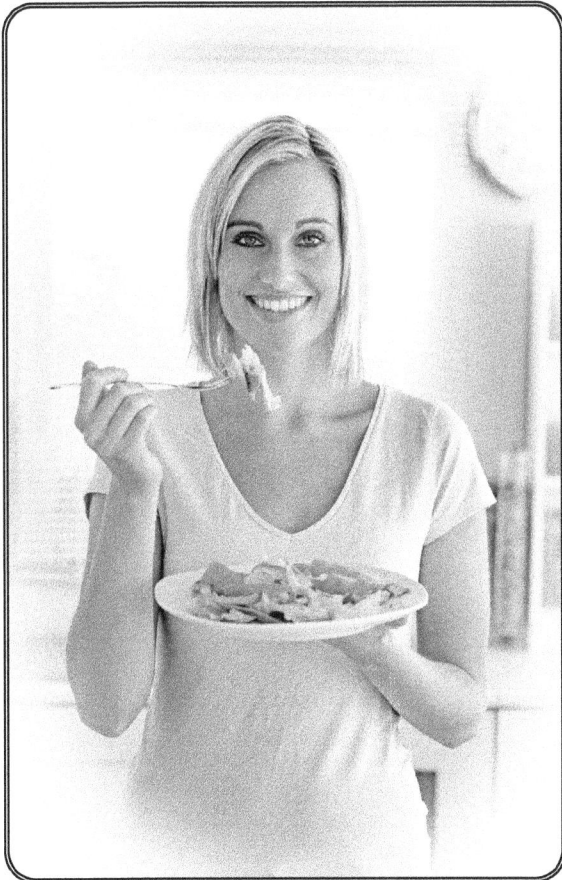

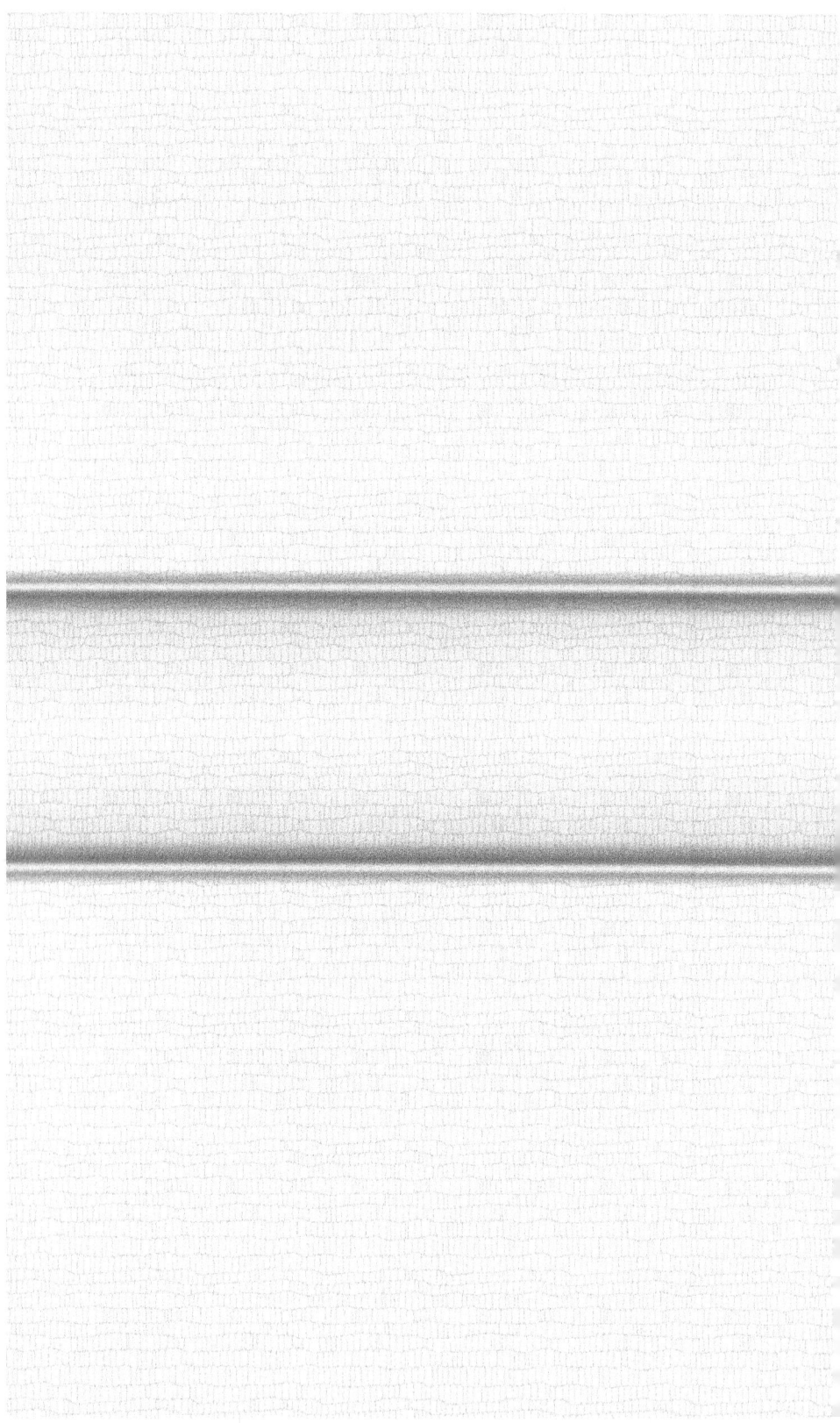

19: Smoothies and Smoothie Bowls

19: Smoothies and Smoothie Bowls

Here are some easy ways to get more than five fruits and vegetables daily.

Smoothies

Best smoothies are made with fruit and vegetables, making adding more fruit and vegetables to your diet fun. Smoothies contain the whole fruit and vegetable, and they provide much-needed fibre. As we know, fibre enhances bowel function and the cleansing process, provides food for the correct bowel flora, encourages good bacteria, helps to balance blood sugar levels, and stops you from feeling hungry.

Smoothies provide nutrients that encourage detoxification, cleansing, regeneration and healing, along with plenty of fresh enzymes that further encourage the process. Here is a list of fruit and vegetables to use in your smoothies, briefly explaining each one's cleansing and healing properties.

Lemon Juice adds a zesty, clean taste. Lemon is renowned for being very alkaline-forming in the body and extremely good for the liver, a major detoxifying organ.

Ginger is often added; it is anti-inflammatory, increases circulation, encourages detoxification and more.

Pineapple is full of enzymes that add cleansing and detoxification, and it is also anti-inflammatory. It is good for digestion.

Passion fruit soothes the digestive tract and is rich in Vitamin C, antioxidants and magnesium. Many people do not get enough magnesium for a functioning bowel, nervous system and muscles.

Blueberries and raspberries are rich sources of antioxidants and are highly cleansing.

Watermelon is perfect for cleansing and hydrating the body; it combats bloating and puffiness.

Cantaloupe melon is rich in antioxidants and beta-carotene, hydrating, and good for healthy mucus membranes, skin and lungs.

Papaya or pawpaw is a potent detoxifier and is crammed with beta-carotene. Papaya contains an enzyme called papain.

Celery helps to cleanse joints, as well as having a diuretic effect that reduces fluid retention. Celery helps to cleanse the body of sodium deposits.

Carrot is an excellent source of beta-carotene (the body converts what it needs to Vitamin A). Carrots are renowned for being good for the liver, a major cleansing organ.

Parsley is a good source of minerals and chlorophyll; it is a powerful cleanser, an excellent blood purifier and is great for stimulating the bowels. Parsley is good for the kidneys and acts as a diuretic, helping to solve fluid retention problems. It reduces coagulants in the veins and helps to clear or prevent kidney stones. Parsley is a very effective cleanser, rich in antioxidants.

Cucumber cleanses the whole system, aids digestion and is a good diuretic (reduces fluid retention). This mild laxative helps flush out the kidneys and the bladder and helps dissolve uric acid buildup.

Courgette (Zucchini) encourages healthy digestion, detoxifies, lowers cholesterol, is a mild laxative and has diuretic properties. Helps the liver to function better, aids the metabolism and helps stabilise blood sugar levels.

Cabbage heals the digestive lining, being rich in vitamin U, which heals ulcers. It is also a very effective cleanser. Use white, red, green, spring and Chinese cabbage (my favourite).

Beetroot is an excellent blood purifier and is helpful for the liver. Some people use it now, but not all like it as a smoothie.

Mango is very good for cleansing and detoxifying, especially the kidneys and the bloodstream. Mango also strengthens and invigorates the nerve tissues, muscles, heart, and other body parts. The fruit cleanses the body and helps the immune system fight infections.

Pumpkin and squash are rich in beta-carotene, a powerful antioxidant that the body uses to convert into vitamin A by the liver. Beta-carotene is excellent for the health of the skin, lungs and bowel lining.

Apples are high in antioxidants, flavonoids and fibre, but particularly a fibre called pectin. All fibre is good at cleansing, but pectin is particularly good for cleansing the colon and flushing toxins out of the system. The high pectin content in apples helps remove cholesterol and toxic metal residues. Apples are particularly good at helping to cleanse the liver and gallbladder, and they contain vitamin C. Apples are a great hedge against constipation, which can be a problem for older people. The old saying that an apple a day keeps the doctor away has more than a grain of truth in it.

Pears are good for thyroid function.

Dark green leaves are good sources of minerals and chlorophyll, powerful cleansers, good blood purifiers, and great for stimulating the bowels. These strengthen the blood, especially for those who are prone to anaemia.

Coconut water is an excellent hydrator.

Plant powders: buy slowly dried at low temperatures.

Acerola berry powder is super high in vitamin C.

Maca powder is rich in calcium, iron and fibre.

Spirulina is super-rich in chlorophyll and essential fatty acids, and renowned for being a natural multi-vitamin & mineral, but in a natural form that is easy to digest and absorb.

Acai Powder is high in fibre, minerals, omega essential fatty acids and antioxidants.

Sea Buckthorn Berry powder, flavour a little like passion fruit. Vitamin C, A, B1, B2, E plus Omega-7.

Protein-Rich Smoothies

Some people want a healthy meal replacer or a protein-rich sports drink, so these smoothies should include some sort of protein. When people think of adding protein to their smoothies, they think of the protein powders in health shops, bodybuilding places or supermarkets. These popular protein sources are whey or soy protein powder, but they can contain some highly processed ingredients, flavourings, natural or artificial sweeteners, chemicals and heavy metals. Whey is unsuitable for Vegans, and too much soya is not a good idea.

There are healthier alternatives, which are powders made from plant protein powders like hemp, brown rice or pea powder, but you need to read the labels very carefully and check out what else the product contains. On the other hand, you can add protein from actual, natural protein-rich foods. So, what can you add to your smoothie that contains protein and is rich in nutrients and fibre? What can you add that is natural and helps to stave off hunger by stabilising blood sugar levels? Or, what would work after some exercise?

Organic natural yoghurt is one, because an ounce contains about seven grams of protein. Yoghurt contains healthy bacteria, but only if it's a real live natural quality Yoghurt and not if you are a vegan or lactose intolerant.

Nuts are another, and there are two ways of adding these, depending on how good your blender is. The first is to add some organic unsweetened almond butter, peanut butter, or other nut butter. If you like tahini (sesame paste), add some of that. One tablespoon of almond butter contains about two grams of protein. One tablespoon of peanut butter contains about three grams of protein. Secondly, take any raw, unsalted nuts and soak them in water the night before, discard the water in the morning and add the soaked nuts to your blender. Soaking them the night before activates enzymes and makes them easier to digest. Soaking them makes it much easier to blend into the smoothie. Two ounces of walnuts contain about four grams of protein, and nuts add essential fatty acids, magnesium and fibre to the system.

Pumpkin Seeds contain about three grams of protein in a tablespoon and are a good source of magnesium, zinc and omega-3s. Pumpkin seeds also contain tryptophan, the sleep-inducing amino acid found in turkey. However, for most people, this just means it helps to calm the nervous system.

Chia Seeds have about four grams of protein per tablespoon. Used for centuries, these are full of fibre, omega-3 fatty acids, and calcium. Soak overnight in water (they will expand and become mucilaginous, like linseeds), then add to your smoothie. I use a lot of chia and flax seeds in various ways, but I never cook them. **Linseeds** (flaxseeds) have about two grams of protein per tablespoon. Soak overnight in some water (they will expand and become mucilaginous, like chia seeds), then add to your smoothie. They are excellent for correcting constipation and for soothing the digestive tract.

Sunflower seeds have about one and a half grams of protein per tablespoon. Sunflower seeds are a good source of copper and vitamin E and are helpful for blood circulation.

Organic oats contain about two-and-a-half grams of protein for two ounces of dry weight. Oats contain soluble fibre that is good for cholesterol, and they are excellent for feeding the nervous system. Soak the oats overnight in some water as this softens the oats, making them easier to blend into a smooth texture, and also stops the oats from expanding in the smoothie.

Coconut flesh is useful, as four ounces contain about two-and-a-half grams of protein, and it tastes so good. Coconut is good for those who suffer from candida because it contains caprylic acid. Coconut can be added in a couple of ways; as unsweetened coconut milk, from a can or a carton, or organic natural unsweetened coconut flakes soaked overnight and added to your blender with all your other ingredients.

Pure organic cocoa powder is surprising, but it contains four grams of protein per ounce, is full of anti-oxidants and happy-making compounds, and of course, it tastes wonderful. Cocoa can be a stimulant, so it is best not to take it late in the day.

A Smoothie Bowl

A thick smoothie is put in a bowl and then topped with various fresh or dried fruits, nuts, seeds etc. The combination is endless. You will need a spoon and bowl instead of a straw and glass because smoothie bowls are eaten, not slurped. Smoothie bowls are healthy, seriously nourishing, easy to digest and blissfully delicious. Of course, it depends on how they are made and the ingredients used.

A smoothie bowl is more filling than a standard smoothie and, indeed, more interesting than a smoothie, and it can be used for breakfast, lunch or a light supper. Take one to work or eat one after a heavy workout. Tempted by dessert? Have a smoothie bowl instead.

Smoothie Bowl Ingredients

You could use fresh and frozen fruit, and vegetables like carrots, beets, cucumber, courgettes, avocado, ginger, and cinnamon.

Avocado – gives the first layer a rich, smooth texture when added to the smoothie. They are rich in folate acid, beta carotene, lutein, iron, zinc, several B vitamins and importantly, fats that are extremely good for us, especially for our hearts.

Yoghurt should be organic, natural, and plain. Don't use any flavoured types of yoghurt, as they contain sugar, sweeteners, and other unhealthful ingredients. Try organic goat or sheep's yoghurt. This is not for you if you are a vegan or lactose intolerant. Do not add dairy products of any kind if you plan to use smoothie bowls for a detox cleanse.

Coconut Yoghurt (use organic) is ideal for anyone who wants to avoid animal products, and it is now so easy to find in some supermarkets.

Plant-based milk: use only natural, unflavoured, and unsweetened:
Almond milk.
Rice milk.
Oat milk.
Hazelnut milk.
Coconut Milk.
Coconut Water.
Seeds – only raw
Pumpkin
Sunflower
Linseeds
Chia
Hemp

Nuts – only raw, either zapped into the smoothie or sprinkled on top.
Walnuts.
Almonds.
Pecan.
Hazelnuts.

Coconut flesh – natural unsweetened.
Organic dried fruit – make sure they are dried without any added sweetness.
Cranberries (no added sugar) contain vitamins A and C, minerals iron and potassium, and plenty of fibre.

Apricots (unsulphured) contain vitamins A, B and C, minerals, iron, magnesium and phosphorus, and plenty of fibre.

Dates – contain vitamins A, B and C and minerals iron, magnesium and phosphorus plus fibre.

Mulberries – contain vitamins C and K, minerals, iron and calcium. Fibre, anthocyanins and resveratrol.

Incan berries – contain vitamins A, B1, B2, B6, B12, C, pectin, bioflavonoids, phosphorus and a small amount of melatonin.

Acai – is high in fibre, minerals, omega essential fatty acids and antioxidants.

Buy sun-dried or those processed at low temperatures retaining an optimum number of nutrients.

Oils (keep in a cool place away from light).
Cold-pressed Coconut Oil – contains lauric acid, capric acid and caprylic acid, which are antimicrobial, antioxidant, anti-fungal and antibacterial. Good for the immune system, proper digestion and regulating metabolism, plus much more.

Other
Oats
Protein powder plant-based vegan, hemp, pea or rice protein.
Chocolate – 100% pure powder.
Natural vanilla extract or vanilla pod – vanilla has a sweet taste and a lovely flavour.
Salt.
Plant powders – buy slowly dried at low temperatures.
Acerola berry – super high in vitamin C.

Maca (Peruvian ginseng) is rich in calcium, iron and fibre.

Spirulina – super-rich in chlorophyll, essential fatty acids, also renowned for being a natural multi-vitamin & mineral. In a natural form that is easy to digest and absorb.

Acai Powder – is high in fibre, minerals, omega essential fatty acids and antioxidants.

Sea Buckthorn Berry – flavour a little like passion fruit. Vitamin C, A, B1, B2, E plus omega-7.

Why buy powders? Some ingredients are not readily available, so you may have to buy powders and add them to your smoothie bowl.

Do Not Use the Following

Sugar.

Honey.

Agave.

Sweeteners.

Syrups of any kind.

Pure granulated fructose (not to be confused with fruit).

Or anything with an "ose" at the end – Sucrose, Lactose, Glucose, Dextrose etc.

If you want your smoothie bowl to be a little sweeter, use a banana, a little dried fruit or some extra fresh fruit. Add a little natural vanilla or cinnamon, which sweeten without adding any sweetener.

Keep your dried produce in air-tight containers in cool, dark places away from light. Or keep some in the fridge and some in the freezer, especially if you buy some ingredients in bulk.

Making Your Smoothie Bowl

The first layer of your smoothie bowl is made with fruit, vegetables, powders, linseeds or chia seeds. You can blend dried oats into the mixture by pouring them in and leaving the mixture to thicken for thirty minutes, or you can use chia seeds or flaxseeds in exactly the same way.

For the second layer, add neat rows of sliced fresh fruit and berries, then make the third layer by sprinkling on chopped nuts and seeds. You can add cocoa powder or crushed cocoa nibs, if you like.

Enjoy eating your smoothie bowl at any time of the day.

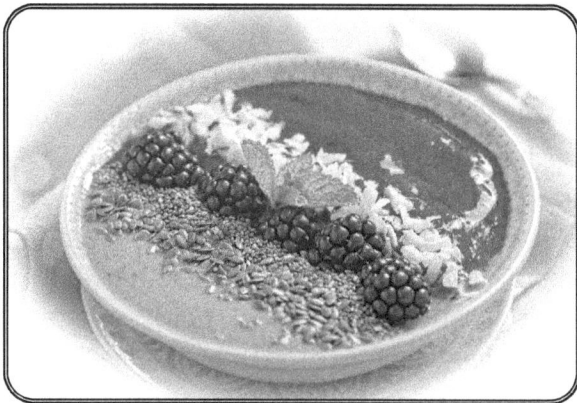

SMOOTHIE BOWL

20: Sprouting, Buddha Bowl or Nourish Bowl

20: Sprouting, Buddha Bowl or Nourish Bowl

Sprouts

It is easy and cheap to produce sprouts yourself in as little as three days, and they are bursting with energy, enzymes and healing properties.

These days, I use large mason 1.5-litre jars with lids especially made for mason jars and sprouting. The lid has tiny holes that are ideal for small seeds. I used a large glass jar in the past, covered the opening with a piece of netting (or similar fabric), and secured it with an elastic band. This works really well, too. The seeds I use are organic alfalfa, beet, radish, broccoli, red clover, lentils and mung beans.

To make sprouts, put approximately three tablespoons of seeds into the jar, cover them with plenty of water and allow them to soak overnight. In the morning, place the lid or cloth over the opening and drain the water. Add more water, rinse the seeds and drain again. Now place the jar on its side, on the countertop in the kitchen near the sink. This is a convenient place that will remind you to rinse them regularly.

The seeds must be rinsed two or three times daily, and all the water must be drained out each time. Do not let the seeds sit in water, as they will rot. The netting or the lid act as a sieve, allowing water in and out without losing any seeds. The rinsing is very important because the seeds could either not grow or go mouldy. Be reasonably careful when rinsing the growing sprouts to avoid damaging them. Depending on the seed and the temperature, they sprout in three to five days.

Once the sprouts are ready, remove them from the jar and place them in a large bowl of water. Move the sprouts around in the water and remove the seed husks, don't worry if you can't remove every single one. Throw the husks away or compost them.

Why sprout? You will have fresh organic food all year round, especially during the winter months. It's much cheaper to do your own sprouting than buying ready-sprouted seeds; it's easy, and your own are so much fresher. They are bursting with nutrients and, importantly, are a rich source of enzymes. These sprouted seeds are at their peak performance, so to speak, enzyme and nutrition-wise. As you will see, the jar method is not the only way to sprout.

You can buy or make sprouting bags from natural organic fabric such as hemp or linen, neither of which will rot. The bags are dunked into the water two or three times daily and then hung up to drain over a sink or tray.

Sprouting trays are made especially for sprouting, and they are perforated to allow water to drip through and air to circulate. The trays are stacked, and the last tray catches all the water.

Spiralized Veggies – Pasta Substitutes

The spiralizer is a simple non-electrical gadget you can find online or an attachment to a food processor. It turns vegetables into spaghetti or noodle shapes. This is another way to eat more vegetables while reducing refined carbohydrates. Any of your favourite pasta sauces can be used with spiralized vegetables instead of your usual spaghetti-shaped pasta. Spiralized vegetables can also replace noodles in your favourite Asian noodle dish, or be used in salads to add more interest in texture and visual variety. Check out recipes for pancakes made from spiralized veggies and spiralized sweet potatoes.

Rice Substitute

You may have seen or used cauliflower rice which is a wonderful substitute for rice, and this is another way to cut down on starch and add more vegetables to your daily amount because it means cutting vegetables to the size of rice grains. Besides cauliflower, you could use broccoli, carrots, beetroot, butternut squash or pumpkin. Cauliflower is the first choice as it looks more like rice than beetroot.

Use the food processor with the blade attachment. Clean the vegetables, chop them into large chunks, and place them into the food processor in batches without adding too many in one go. Zap the vegetables carefully until they are the consistency and size of rice.

Invest in some recipe books. I am lucky to have a place near me called the Book Barn; it's enormous and full of excellent second-hand books. Get books that show you how to incorporate more vegetables into your week in inviting and interesting ways.

Buddha Bowl or Nourish Bowl

This another way to eat more vegetables in a healthy, interesting and tasty way. About five years ago, Australia introduced the Buddha Bowl or Nourish Bowl and Poke Bowl, which became trendy in restaurants. I lived in Australia for four years and can attest to their amazingly fresh and healthy foods, even twenty years ago. These dishes are a meal in a bowl, but it's more interesting than it sounds. Delicious, fresh, nutritious food can come in many combinations that are never boring and always colourful and appealing. There is a simple basic formula to them.

Buddha Bowls or Nourish Bowls, also known as Hippie Bowls or Macro Bowls, consist of Vegetarian and Vegan food. The Poke Bowl was originally from Hawaii and contained thinly sliced raw tuna with rice and other fresh ingredients. They can be eaten any time, morning, noon or night. Served cold or hot.

Nourish Bowls are rich in antioxidants, vitamins and minerals, and enzymes. They are easy on digestion, increase metabolism, boost immunity, and balance cholesterol levels. Generally, a bowl contains five key categories:

A grain (quinoa, millet or brown rice).
A legume (bean or lentil).
Vegetables, such as roasted vegetables, fresh vegetables or sprouts.
A sauce or dressing.
Nuts and seeds.

Some people want to add protein to their Buddha bowls, such as fish, chicken, or meat.

These bowls make a great way to load up on veggies for lunch at work or during a busy day when you don't have time to prepare a healthy lunch or breakfast, and they are easy to transport in one dish with a lid, which makes them convenient, nutritious and economical.

Grains
For convenience, cook a batch of one of the grains mentioned above. If you are in a hurry, pick quinoa which is much quicker to cook than brown rice. Store in a fridge for up to four days.

Beans

Here you have choices; either buy tinned beans and lentils, or cook your own. Dried beans need soaking overnight, and you must throw the water away in the morning. Add fresh water and cook for about two hours. Make a large batch and put some in the freezer. Lentils cook in much less time.

Protein

(Not vegan or vegetarian). Add cooked salmon, tinned tuna, smoked trout, boiled eggs, cold chicken and leftover Sunday roast meat.

Oven-roast sliced sweet potato, yellow or red peppers, mushrooms and onions. Place on a tray, brush with some olive oil and roast them in a moderate oven until soft. Once cooled, place in the fridge in an airtight container. I have purchased a lot of different-sized glass containers that come with clip-on plastic lids as I prefer to keep food in glass rather than plastic.

Fresh Vegetables

Grate carrots and courgettes, dice cooked beetroot and fresh cucumber, and slice tomato and radishes.

You could add fresh fruit like sliced mango, apple or pear, depending on the other ingredients and dressing of your Nourish bowl that day.

A Simple Dressing

Choose organic apple cider vinegar, extra virgin oil, fresh herbs, salt and pepper.

Avocado Dressing
Select a ripe avocado, add lemon or lime juice to taste, a small bunch of fresh coriander, about 170 grammes of yoghurt, oat cream or almond milk, plus two spring onions and salt to taste. Place in a blender and zap until smooth.

Tahini Sauce
115g of tahini, two dried pitted dates, the juice of one small-sized fresh lemon, three tablespoons of water or more to give the consistency you want and blend in a blender, then add salt and pepper to taste.

Peanut Butter Sauce
Add equal amounts of peanut butter to water, a one-inch piece of fresh ginger, two or three pitted dried dates and apple cider vinegar. Blend until smooth.

Yoghurt Dressing
Natural yoghurt, mixed fresh herbs and a small garlic clove (optional).

Apple Dressing
One or two large apples, peeled and cored, a piece of ginger, lemon juice to taste, apple cider vinegar, extra virgin oil, salt and pepper. Place all ingredients into a blender and blend until smooth. A pear would work well too.

Cashew Nut Creamy Dressing
One cup of unsalted cashew nuts soaked overnight (throw the water away in the morning), add a third of a cup of fresh water, and add one tablespoon of apple cider vinegar, salt

and pepper. Place all the ingredients into a blender and zap until smooth and creamy.

Temperature - remember these bowls can be eaten hot, warm or cold at home, and then the leftovers are put in the fridge for another day.

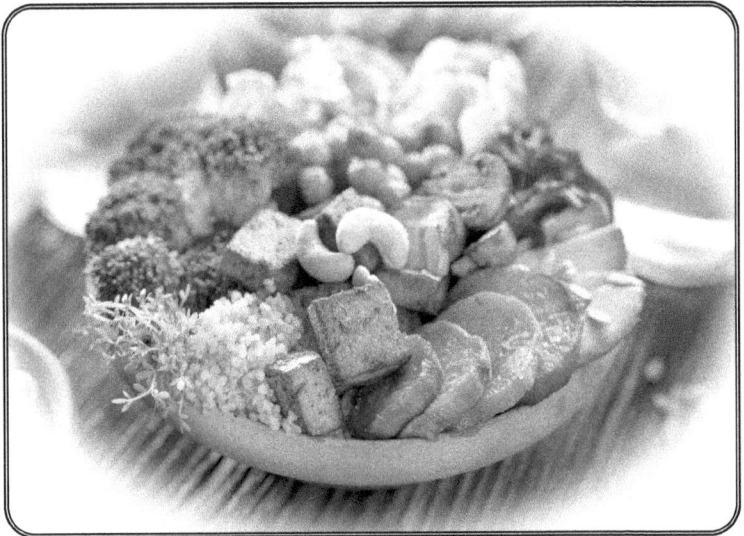

BUDDHA BOWL

21: Fasting and Unusual Diets

21: Fasting and Unusual Diets

Fasting

Some people believe in doing without food for long periods, either because they have little appetite and prefer to live on coffee and cigarettes, or because they spend their days running around at work and only eat in the evening and at weekends. Some hate eating in front of others (those with the sun, moon or ascendant in Scorpio are often like this), and some people endeavour to control their weight by going without food for a day or two each week.

Some fast for religious reasons. The Yom Kippur fast is a good example because not only do orthodox Jews avoid food for twenty-four hours, but they don't drink water or even brush their teeth in case something inadvertently goes down their throats! Religious Muslims observe a month of Ramadan where they don't eat until the sun goes down each day, while Christians restrict their diets during Lent, avoiding alcohol, treats, meat and much else. Salvationists call this "the time of self-denial". Others fast for a day or two as a penance for some supposed sin or to bring them closer to God. All this is fine if it focuses your mind and makes you happy, but it shouldn't be carried too far.

All the studies done by Slimming World, Diabetes UK and other such good organisations show that eating regular meals comprising sensible food is the answer to staying slim and fit. I feel that as long as you are healthy, an occasional day without food won't hurt as long as you drink plenty of water while fasting.

Vegetarianism or Veganism

These food choices are becoming popular, and they don't seem to hurt those living that way, so maybe we don't need animal products. However, this is a personal choice and not something that should be imposed on those who don't want to give up the omnivorous life.

It doesn't matter whether you choose to be a vegan, a vegetarian, a carnivore, or all of them some of the time, as all diets can be healthy or unhealthy, and the choice is entirely up to you. The most important thing, first and foremost, is that your diet includes a lot of fresh vegetables and fruit daily, along with other healthy quality products.

Every decade sees new diets enter the arena, with many people rushing to try them as soon as they discover them, usually for weight-loss reasons. They all come and go from the `F-plan to the Atkins diet. We currently have the Paleo and Keto diets; the keto diet is similar to the old Atkins diet, intending to establish ketosis, thus burning fat for energy. Two diets have been around for decades, and in some societies for hundreds of years. For many people, they are a way of life rather than just a diet, and these are the vegan and vegetarian diets.

The vegan diet has become ever more popular in the last decade as more and more people have decided to give up animal products for ethical, environmental or health reasons (that last bit, of course, depends on how a vegan diet is approached). Many vegans also avoid clothing made from wool or leather.

When done right, veganism is healthy and better for the environment. When poorly done, it can increase the risk of nutritional deficiencies. Vegans find all animal exploitation unacceptable, whether for food, clothing, or beauty, so they avoid lanolin wax from sheep or beeswax, or supplements like velvet from deer antlers or royal jelly from bees.

A vegan way of life means no animal products whatsoever, avoiding eggs, butter, milk, cheese, yoghurt, meat, suet, fish, seafood, honey, royal jelly, whey, casein and gelatine. It includes plenty of plant-based foods like fruit, vegetables, nuts, seeds, legumes (lentils and beans) and whole grains.

Variations on a vegan diet are within the realms of veganism, so it's all down to what works for the individual. The main one is based on a wide variety of whole plant foods such as fruits, vegetables, whole grains, legumes, nuts and seeds, cooked and raw.

Another variation is the raw diet based on raw fruits, vegetables, nuts, seeds or plant foods cooked below 118°F (48°C), which helps preserve more nutrients and enzymes. Eighty-ten-ten is a raw-food vegan diet that is low in fat from fat-rich plants such as nuts and avocados and is more reliant on raw fruits and soft greens instead. Also known as the low-fat, raw-food vegan diet or fruitarian diet, this comprises eighty per cent carbs from raw vegetables and raw fruit, ten per cent from protein nuts and seeds and ten per cent from fats.

Then there is the low-fat, high-carb vegan diet similar to the 80/10/10, which includes cooked starches like potatoes, brown rice and organic corn.

"Raw until four" is a low-fat vegan diet. Only raw foods until four in the afternoon; after that, there is the option to have cooked, plant-based foods.

Junk-food vegan processed foods are now readily available in many supermarkets. Is this a good idea?

A vegetarian diet means no meat or fish but does include eggs, butter, milk, yoghurt, cheese and honey. Some people who want to give up meat for animal welfare, environmental or health reasons find being a vegan too difficult and opt to be a vegetarian. I know people who vacillate between being a vegetarian and a vegan. That's fine; there are no rules, and it's up to you - there are no diet police.

Whether you are a vegan, vegetarian or carnivore, or if a health problem means avoiding gluten, things are so much easier today than ever before. For instance, I can't eat many eggs, so when I want to bake, I use chia and flaxseeds, which are ideal for egg replacement. To replace one egg, simply mix one tablespoon of chia or ground flaxseeds with three tablespoons of hot water and allow it to rest until it thickens. For two eggs, use two tablespoons of seeds, six of hot water, and so on.

Cow's milk substitutes such as coconut, almond and oat milk are everywhere. Coconut or goat's Yoghurt exists. Gluten-free baking and products have come a long way since the early days.

Note from Sasha, the editor…
People treated for cancer can become intolerant of gluten, wheat or dairy products for a year or two after Chemotherapy or even permanently. As about half the population will have some form of cancer sooner or later, this is becoming common. On a personal note, I have always been somewhat intolerant of eggs, so I will try the chia and flaxseed solution for cooking and see how that goes. Thanks, Sonia

---

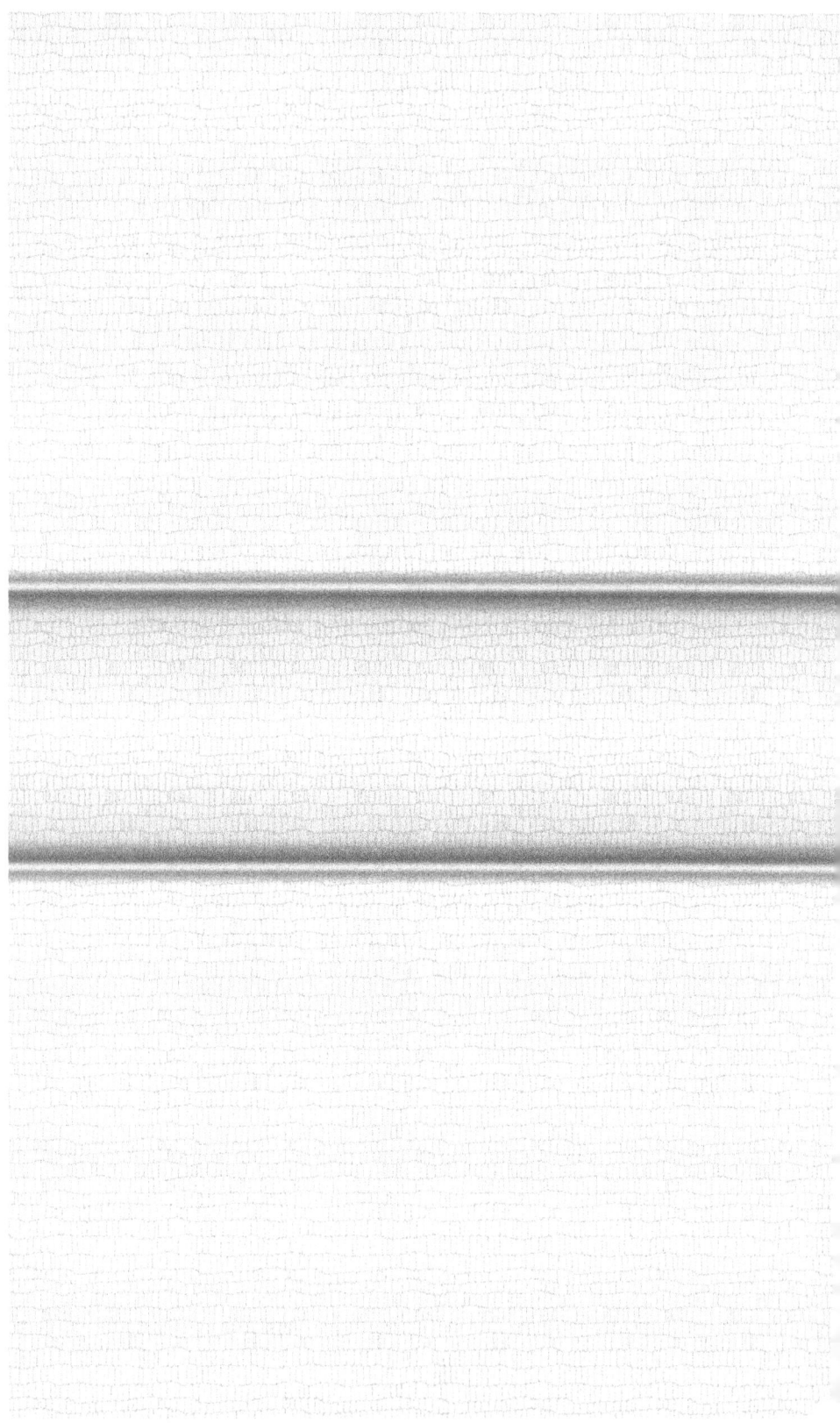

22: The Shopping List

22: The Shopping List

Protein
Free-range or organic if possible.
Beef – most acid-forming.
Lamb.
Chicken.
Duck.
Venison.
Turkey.
Fish - wild if possible.
Eggs – organic.
Goat's cheese - not matured too long (if no dairy problem).
Natural Goat's plain Yoghurt (if no dairy problem).
Beans or lentils mixed with grains (for a complete protein).

Only eat meat items that are obvious, such as steak, roasting meats, lamb chops, chicken and so on. Avoid processed meats such as sausages, sausage rolls, hot dogs, deli meats and meat pies.

Nuts and Seeds.
Raw nuts and seeds – good source of essential fatty acids, fibre and protein.
Almonds.

Walnuts.
Sesame seeds.
Flaxseeds (Linseeds).
Hemp seeds.
Chia Seeds.
Cashews.
Sunflower seeds.
Pumpkin seeds.
Other raw unsalted nuts.

Fresh Fruit and Vegetables.
Lots of them, in as wide a variety as possible.

Grains & Seeds - Only Whole Grains.
Oats.
Millet.
Quinoa.
Brown rice.
Spelt.
Kamut.
Buckwheat.
Amaranth.
Corn - only organic.

Sweetening – in Moderation
Dried fruit.
Honey.
Molasses.
Maple syrup.
Stevia.

Drinks
Water.

Herbal teas.
Smoothies – made with whole fruit and vegetable.
Green Tea.
Alcohol – occasionally.

Pasta
Rice noodles.
Soba noodles made from 100% buckwheat.
Invest in a spiralizer. A gadget that cut my vegetables into long, thin spirals. I use this instead of grain pasta with pesto sauce.

General Items
Organic apple cider vinegar.
Quality Salt - I use Celtic and Anglesey salt.
Black Pepper Corn - freshly ground when needed.
Organic stock cubes - msg-free, additive-free, gluten-free.
All Herbs.
All Spices.
All Beans.
All Lentils.
Rice Milk.
Oat Milk.
Almond Milk.
Brown Rice.
Tahini (sesame butter).
Butter (no margarine).

Sprouting
Mung beans.
Lentils.
Grains.
All beans – except red beans and soybeans.

Oils

Extra virgin, cold-pressed, expelled or first pressed.
Olive oil.
Sesame oil - for stir-fries.
Coconut oil - best on the list for heating.
Walnut oil.
Hemp oil.
Flaxseed oil.

Treats

70% to 80% cocoa chocolate.
Dried fruit.
Natural organic popcorn.
Natural nut butter like almond.
Fresh fruit.
Raw nuts and seeds.

Your Food Store

Clean out your kitchen store cupboards and fridge occasionally, and throw out everything that is out-of-date. Finding what's lurking at the back of the cupboard is always a surprise. Decide what other foods would be better removed, read the labels carefully and check all ingredients. Don't be tempted to keep unhealthy ingredients. It can be a case of starting again, ensuring your food store and fridge are stocked with healthy food. If budget is a problem, do this gradually, starting with out-of-date products and gradually replacing other food items.

Useful Swaps

On the next page is a quick guide with some easy swaps.

Nutrition in Focus

Original Food Item	Healthy Choice Item
White rice	Brown rice
Rice	Cauliflower and veg rice
Couscous	Millet or quinoa
White bread	Wholemeal, spelt, sourdough rye, gluten-free
Spread	Butter
Spaghetti	Wholemeal or buckwheat soba spaghetti
Sugar	Dried fruit, honey, mashed banana
Salt	Anglesey or Himalayan salt
Vegetable oil	Extra virgin or coconut oil
Flavoured yoghurt	Natural live yoghurt
snacks	Fruit and nuts
Shop bought smoothies	Homemade smoothies
Salty nuts	Raw nuts
Cows cheese	Goat or sheep cheese
White flour	Wholemeal, buckwheat, coconut, gram
Cream	Natural live yoghurt
Milk chocolate	Dark organic chocolate
Soft drinks	Water, sparkling water, or water infused with fruit or kombucha
Coffee	Lemon or herbal tea
Cereal	Fresh fruit, natural Yoghurt sprinkled with oats, nuts and seeds. Organic eggs with leftover vegetables
Potatoes	Sweet potatoes
Chips	Baked or boiled new potatoes

Conclusion

Conclusion

Eating well is fundamental to living an active life with fewer ailments that can turn into chronic conditions. Read labels very carefully, and be mindful of when you eat and how you eat. Making changes can be daunting, and breaking habits can be difficult. So where to start? See it as a step-by-step process and tackle some of the easier things first; this, of course, is different for each person. Set goals at the beginning of each week, and don't beat yourself up if you don't achieve all of them, as it takes time to make changes. Eat better, do some exercise and rest when you can. It all makes perfect sense.

Good luck,

Sonia

Index

Index

Index

Index

Index

Index

www.ingramcontent.com/pod-product-compliance
Lightning Source LLC
Chambersburg PA
CBHW042120190326
41519CB00031B/7561